Psychopharmacology for Nonpsychiatrists

Daniel P. Greenfield

Psychopharmacology for Nonpsychiatrists

A Primer

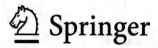 Springer

Daniel P. Greenfield
Clinical Professor of Neuroscience (Psychiatry)
Seton Hall University
Short Hills
NJ
USA

ISBN 978-3-030-82509-6   ISBN 978-3-030-82507-2   (eBook)
https://doi.org/10.1007/978-3-030-82507-2

This Springer imprint is published by the registered company Springer Nature Switzerland AG
The registered company address is: Gewerbestrasse 11, 6330 Cham, Switzerland

As with my previous volumes, this Primer *is dedicated to my family, children, and grandchildren (now six of them!), and to the colleagues, students, and friends who shared their interests and experiences with me over the years, and gave me the database for this book.*

– Daniel P. Greenfield

Clinical Foreword

After years of teaching in a physician assistant (PA) program, I am gradually coming to the conclusion that the undergraduate coursework premedical programs require of their students may be doing a disservice in preparing these students for their training program. An unfortunate consequence of heavy basic science preparation is that it can lead to very "black and white" thinking. By the time students finish a chemistry course, they can determine precisely what will be synthesized when a mole of compound A is added to a mole of compound B. At the conclusion of a physics course, students can calculate to the millimeter where a projectile will land. Students master this coursework and eagerly move on to their medical training. It does not take long for these students to realize that people are extraordinarily, biologically complex.

Mental and behavioral health—and the associated neuroscience—present a special challenge to a clinician in training. Many pathologic processes in medicine are fairly understandable and certain diagnoses can be arrived at using cultures and biopsies, and the mechanisms for medications like analgesics and antibiotics are generally readily understood. However, diagnosis and treatment in psychiatry and mental and behavioral health can often seem mysterious. Diagnostic criteria are fluid, and medication regimens can be complex with effects only becoming apparent over the course of weeks.

Thus, the need for this *Primer*.

Dr. Daniel Greenfield has proven to be a talented educator in the almost two decades he has been involved in teaching psychiatry and mental and behavioral health to PA students. His coursework is devoted less to conveying facts and more toward inculcating a manner of clinical reasoning and thinking in students. Psychopharmacology is frequently a single topic among many covered at a lightning pace during a pharmacology course. His latest effort will provide valuable additional foundational information for students who wish to cultivate a deeper understanding of an often-mysterious medication family.

This book helpfully locates psychopharmacology within the larger context of psychiatric treatment and briefly discusses the variety of therapeutic and somatic techniques available to providers and their patients. In addition, since many patients with psychiatric conditions unfortunately find themselves interacting with the justice system, Dr. Greenfield concludes with useful considerations related to the intersection of mental health and the law.

Many areas of the country are experiencing an acute shortage of mental healthcare providers. This shortage is greatly exacerbated by the opioid abuse crisis and the COVID-19 pandemic our nation faces. Primary care providers will increasingly find themselves in a position of needing to initiate and monitor psychopharmacologic therapy. Dr. Greenfield's extensive experience has allowed him to create an easily readable book that will serve as a welcome information source as these clinicians work to develop a sound therapeutic plan for their troubled patients.

June, 2020   Christopher J. Hanifin
                                               Chairperson and Program Director
                                                   Physician Assistant Program
                                                       Seton Hall University
                                                        South Orange, NJ
                                                                USA

Legal/Forensic Foreword

This latest work by Dr. Daniel Greenfield on psychopharmacology is a must read for any person involved in the legal system in any capacity whether judge, lawyer, litigant, or party. I have been engaged in the legal system for almost 50 years as an attorney, judge and currently as full-time faculty in justice at a university. My professional experience, particularly as a trial Judge for over 27 years, provides me a unique perspective of the value, necessity, and need to have a forensic psychiatric expert who possesses the education, expertise, forensic qualifications, and "real-world" experience to render a credible opinion on the effect of drug use on civil or family law cases.

I have known Dr. Greenfield professionally for over two decades. We have interacted in cases when he testified in my court as a psychiatric expert to the competence, sanity, or insanity of a defendant in cases. I have attended his presentations on "Forensic Science and Psychiatry" and, upon retiring from the bench, as co-panelist discussing mental health legal issues for the benefit of members of the legal profession.

His vast experience can be shared once again by reading this wonderfully comprehensive *Primer* that gives invaluable knowledge and insight to any person involved in court cases concerning psychopharmacological and mental capacity issues. He clearly presents an overview of drug use in court cases with great clarity, while also providing a roadmap for the basic questions to ask when selecting an expert. He explains how to assess the appropriate expert's true knowledge of the subject of the case. He does this by giving examples and suggestions of what questions to ask the proposed expert.

The author's research then statistically enumerates types and numbers of cases in which psychopharmacology issues are mentioned, relating these statistics to issues in civil and family court cases. Next, he expertly explains the various ways legal issues manifest themselves in particular cases. The author's unparalleled research provides the reader with statistically concise information on the effect of a multitude of identified substances in different types of court cases, which is of inestimable value to one involved in or studying such litigation. This book provides insight into the possible impact on a court case by psychopharmacological, psychopharmacotherapy, and psychiatric issues raised in a variety of court cases.

Additionally, this well-respected doctor provides definitions and statistics that break down the most complex issues with clarity for a layperson to understand when addressing the difficult problems of legal insanity, diminished capacity, and other mental health problems.

I highly recommend this *Primer* as a marvelous, must-have resource that will guide one through the various issues as explained by a psychiatrist who possesses 40 years of experience not only as a highly respected academician but as a widely recognized forensic expert witness.

June, 2020

Kevin G. Callahan
Superior Court of New Jersey (Hudson Vicinage),
Professor of Criminal Justice
Saint Peter's University
Jersey City, NJ
USA

About the Cover

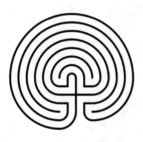 This book's cover is a stylized version of an ancient Cretan labyrinth, or "maze." When the Bronze Age site at Knossos was excavated by explorer Arthur Evans, the complexity of the architecture prompted him to suggest that the palace had been the Labyrinth of Daedalus. Evans found a depiction of a labrys carved into the walls. On the strength of a passage in the Iliad, it has been suggested that the palace was the site of a dancing-ground made for Ariadne by the craftsman Daedalus, where young men and women, of the age of those sent to Crete as prey for the Minotaur, would dance together. By extension, in popular legend, the palace is associated with the myth of the Minotaur. As we also learn from Greek mythology, the labyrinth is a puzzling place, originally the work of the fabled architect Daedalus. The labyrinth's purpose, which Daedalus built for King Minos of Crete, was as a prison in which to hold the monstrous Minotaur.

Our cover's labyrinth symbolizes the convoluted and oft-times confusing path to find and subdue the demon lurking in the mind of a patient or client.

By elongating the shape of the original labyrinth, we also convey a lateral view of the human brain.

Additionally, the Greek key symbol was derived from the labyrinth design and evokes the twists and turns of the river of life.

All in all, walking that winding path to find and understand the best remedies for a mind in distress is a noble and important work. We hope that this *Primer* can help you find your way on that journey.

Author's Disclaimer

I have attempted to ensure that the information, details, facts, and discussions contained in this book are accurate and up to date as of the time of its publication, and consistent with applicable clinical practice and practice standards. However, pharmacology, psychopharmacology, and clinical practice generally are dynamic fields, constantly changing and advancing, so that particular points in this *Primer* may not apply in a particular case or cases. For these reasons, the reader is encouraged to supplement their knowledge by consulting applicable sources and references, including books, textbooks, articles, monographs, electronic databases (such as the *Physician's Desk Reference*, or the *PDR*), other Internet sources, and other such resources. A number of such sources are given in the Selected References section of this *Primer*, as well as other references and sources cited in this book.

In that context, in the three legal/forensic chapters (Chaps. 10, 11, and 12) especially, the information conveyed should not be construed or taken as legal advice, which, not being an attorney or legal professional, the author is not competent to give, and which can be given only by a licensed attorney or qualified legal professional.

Preface

During the time I am writing this Preface, the world is struggling with the COVID-19 pandemic crisis of 2020. We all hope that when the crisis is over, the world will return to "normal" (whatever that is!), and that this crisis, or another such cataclysm, will not happen again.

But for this book, that fact and the age of the author of this book are relevant in two ways:

1. During the COVID-19 crisis, we did less. Less travel, less complex entertainment, less activity, less congregating, less consumption, and the like. A regression, in a way, to slower and simpler times. The obvious exceptions to this observation were those who had to work in dangerous conditions: first responders and direct-care healthcare professionals; food production and service workers; and the workers in the facilities, shops, and stores which provided essential products and services to consumers.
2. In my 40-plus years of clinical practice, and historically before that, I have seen the evolution of psychiatric practice and psychopharmacology through several dramatic quasi-paradigm shifts. I have seen organized psychiatry's view of itself and the public's view of the profession change dramatically. And, of late, those views of the profession have become intertwined with their views of psychopharmacology (or, more properly, "psychopharmacotherapy," as discussed later in this book).

Concerning point (1), the notion of "doing more with less," as we will see in the practical notion of a conservative and minimalist approach to psychopharmacology expressed in this book and in the "deprescribing" climate of today, is being learned in the COVID-19 crisis. This lesson will likely prove to be a useful global cautionary tale. The lesson from this metaphor for psychopharmacology, likewise, is "do more with less." That lesson will be an ongoing theme throughout this book.

In addition, the COVID-19 experience has been extremely anxiety-producing and depressing for almost everybody, including those directly exposed to the virus on a daily basis (health-care workers, food delivery and other transportation workers, pharmacy workers, and other essential workers) and everyone else, most quarantined for long periods of time at home, with many working remotely at their jobs and many who have lost their jobs due to the restrictions of the pandemic. The "Household Pulse Survey" of the National Center for Health Statistics (NCHS) of the Centers for Disease Control and Prevention (CDC), for example, identified an increase of over 30% in psychological symptomatology—including anxiety, depression, or mixed symptoms—compared to the same time period in 2019. This increase was attributed to the many and varied effects of the COVID-19 pandemic: psychological, economic, family-related, occupational, and others (National Center for Health Statistics. [June, 2020]. Anxiety and Depression: Household Pulse Survey. In *Centers for Disease Control and Prevention*. https://www.cdc.gov/nchs/covid19/pulse/mental-health.htm).

Since this increase in psychiatric morbidity will undoubtedly herald an increase in individuals seeking mental health evaluation and treatment; since many of the readers of this book will be sought for that evaluation and treatment; and since psychotropic medications are one of the main tools available to these front line mental health care providers, it is hoped that this book can be a help to those providers as they respond to the influx of new, current, and past patients/clients brought by the COVID-19 pandemic and its aftermath.

Concerning point (2), broadly speaking, five historical trends and positions for psychiatry may be identified in psychiatry over about the past 150 years (recognizing that psychiatry got its start in medieval times through dealing with witchcraft, asylums, often cruel and punishing detention and warehousing of the chronic and serious mentally ill). They are: (1) The strongly neurobiologically based, "organic" psychiatry of Emil Kraepelin ("Dementia Praecox") and Eugen Bleuler ("the schizophrenias"), an era during which neurologists and psychiatrists were closely linked, later drifting apart, and currently coming back together; (2) The classical psychoanalytic and psychotherapy-based approach in the first half of the twentieth century;[1] (3) The "anti-psychiatry" movement beginning in the 1960s and to some extent, continuing to the present day; (4) The ascent and dominance of psychopharmacology in mental health practice and psychiatry also beginning in the 1960s, peaking only recently; and leading to (5) The "deprescribing" movement beginning in the 2010s which is, and in the view of this author and others, currently significantly gaining momentum.

Table P.1 (p. xvii) summarizes these five trends.

---

[1] In this vein, the often-quoted, somewhat paraphrased, words of Harvard Medical School/Massachusetts General Hospital child psychiatrist and Professor of Psychiatry, Leon Eisenberg, MD, in about 1995 ring true: "Let's not allow the brainlessness of psychiatry in the 1930s through 1950s be replaced with the mindlessness of psychiatry in the 1980s and 1990s…"

Table P.1 Historical trends in psychiatry, ca. 1850-present

Time frame	Trend
1. ca. 1850–1900	"Organic" neuropsychiatry of Kaepelin and Bleuler
2. ca. 1900–1950	Classical psychoanalytic/psychodynamic psychiatry
3. ca. 1960–1970s and beyond	"Anti-psychiatry" movement of Szasz, Laing, Scheff, and others
4. ca. 1960-present	"Monotherapy," then "Polypharmacy;" eclipse of psychotherapy and counseling in psychiatric practice
5. Current (2020)	"Deprescribing" movement

The foregoing leads logically to the question "Why write (or read) yet another textbook of psychopharmacology?"

The answer is straightforward. It recognizes and accepts that the professional literature in psychopharmacology is awash with encyclopedic and scholarly tomes and articles, in turn abounding in information, details, protocols, flow charts, data, tables, figures, studies, and the like. These sources provide incredibly detailed and often unnecessary, inapplicable, or even untranslatable information for the practitioner working with, say, anxious and/or depressed patients—the "common colds" of psychiatry.

Therefore, the answer to the question posed above is that this present *Primer* is intended for: (1) The prescribing "front-line" practitioner, including Physician Assistant (PA); Advanced Practice Nurse/Nurse Practitioner (APN/NP); Psychologist with prescribing privileges (in a jurisdiction in which that occurs), and other such professionals, this book is intended as a practical and useful guide applicable to their practices; (2) Other mental health professionals, counselors, therapists, and practitioners who do not themselves prescribe, but whose patients/clients are prescribed psychotropic medications by others, or might benefit from them, this book is intended as a guide to psychopharmacology and "psychopharmacotherapy" (i.e., the therapeutic use of psychopharmacologic agents and medications); (3) Teachers, educators, and academic/school administrators whose students and staff may need mental health evaluations and/or treatment, and/or who might benefit from such evaluations and/or treatment; (4) Nonpsychiatric physicians or dentists whose practices, as many do, involve psychopharmacotherapy; (5) Prescribing health care professionals—such as naturopaths, homeopaths, physical therapists, occupational therapists, speech/language therapists, recreation therapists, and many others—this book is intended as a concise practical guide to psychopharmacology for their patients/clients who are currently on psychotropic drugs or who might benefit from psychopharmacotherapy; (6) Legal and other professionals who are not themselves healthcare professionals, but who interact with healthcare professionals, this book is intended to provide a practical and user-friendly basic understanding of psychopharmacology and psychopharmacotherapy; and (7) Students and trainees in all of these areas and professions, this book is intended as a concise guide and practical handbook of psychopharmacology and psychopharmacotherapy. The only healthcare professionals for whom

Table P.2 The intended audience for this *Primer*

Prescribing "first-line" practitioners: APNs/NPs, PAs, prescriptive-privileged psychologists, others

Non-prescribing mental health professionals whose patients/clients are on (or might benefit from) psychotropic medications (psychologists, social workers, LPCs, other counsellors, drug/alcohol counsellors, pastoral counsellors/hospital chaplains)

Educators (Special Education teachers; classroom teachers; school principals and administrators; Child Study Team members) with students and/or colleagues on psychotropic medications

Non-psychiatric physicians or dentists whose patients/clients are on (or might benefit from) psychotropic medications

Non-prescribing healthcare professionals (chiropractors, PTs, OTs, SLPs [speech and language pathologists], social workers, LPCs, other counsellors, hospital chaplains, RTs [recreation therapists]) whose patients/clients are on (or might benefit from) psychotropic medications

Administrators, legal professionals, and other non-healthcare professionals whose work involves interactions with healthcare professionals

Students and trainees in all of these areas

this present book is *not* intended are practicing and research psychiatrists, and psychiatry trainees (residents). However, medical students interested in psychiatry would likely find this book a useful vade mecum and examination preparation book.

Table P.2 (p. xviii) summarizes the individuals for whom this book is intended.

This *Primer* is organized in four parts, as also indicated in its Table of Contents:

Part I, "Essentials of Psychopharmacology and Psychopharmacotherapy," is the "Basic Principles of Pharmacology, Psychopharmacology, and Psychopharmacotherapy" (Chap. 2); "The Four 'Major Anti-s'" (Chap. 3); "The Sixteen 'Minor Anti-s'" (Chap. 4); "Illicit Substances and Drugs" (Chap. 5); and "Botanicals, Herbals, Nutraceuticals, and (Dietary) Supplements ("Natural Products")" (Chap. 6).

Part II, "Therapies That May Involve Psychopharmacology/Psychopharmacotherapy," provides a succinct overview of selected and representative types of psychotherapy and counseling in contemporary psychiatry and psychology. This Part is geared toward all of the potential readers of this book. The chapters in this Part recognize that, despite the current psychiatric orientation toward largely psychopharmacologic treatment in psychiatric practice, there is more to "psychopharmacotherapy" than simply "pharmacology." The orientation endorsed in this book is toward a conservative and minimalist approach to psychopharmacotherapy, and that "putting the therapy back into psychopharmacotherapy" (S.L. Feder, private communication, 1979) is a worthwhile goal. "An Overview of Therapies in Mental Health Care" (Chap. 7) introduces the two broad categories of psychotherapeutic treatment in psychology, specifically "psychological" and "somatic," and outlines subcategories of treatment within those two broad categories. "Psychotherapies and Counseling" (Chap. 8) and "Somatic Therapies (Somatotherapies)" (Chap. 9) present and discuss examples of those types of treatment.

Recognizing that no prescribing practitioner can be "all things to all people," this book, and this Part in particular, address referrals and consultations for non-pharmacotherapeutic interventions from a variety of practitioners and professionals. The emphasis throughout this *Primer*, in that vein, is on interdisciplinary and holistic treatment approaches to individuals with the conditions and concerns presented and discussed in this book.

Part III, "Forensic and Legal Applications of Psychopharmacology/ Psychopharmacotherapy," draws on this author's long experience in various aspects of forensic psychiatry and recognizes both the extent and usefulness of knowledge on a legal professional's part of psychopharmacotherapy in its myriad potential applications in the law. "Overview" (Chap. 10) gives a survey of these applications. "Selection and Use of Experts: Five Questions" (Chap. 11) and "Evaluating Versus Treating Doctor/Therapist: A Word to the Wise" (Chap. 12) both focus on practical and sometimes problematic areas that frequently occur for trial attorneys and legal professionals generally.

Part IV, "Synthesis and Conclusions" (Chap. 13), pulls together salient points reviewed in this book in order to assist the reader in the practical psychopharmacotherapeutic treatment of patients/clients.

Last, for the purposes of this Preface, I emphasize that this *Primer* is *not* intended as a comprehensive or encyclopedic research or reference source, or as a guide or cookbook for actual prescribing of the psychotropic medications discussed in the *Primer*. For that purpose and for such detailed information, the reader is directed to the applicable detailed Selected References listed at the end of this Preface. I also reemphasize two points made in the Author's Disclaimer earlier in this book, namely that (1) Although I have attempted to ensure accuracy and current information in this *Primer*, in the rapidly-changing field of psychopharmacology, some information will necessarily be outdated by the time this volume is published. The interested and questioning reader is advised and encouraged to supplement or expand their information from this *Primer* by consulting the Selected References, comparable works, electronic databases, Internet sources, and the like; and (2) Since this book is also *not* intended as a textbook or manual for the psychopharmacotherapeutic treatment and management of patients/clients with psychiatric disorders, the reader is also advised to consult their healthcare professional/treatment provider for treatment advice. Similarly, this *Primer* does not purport to provide formal legal advice or counsel, which can only be given by a qualified legal professional.

A Note On References

Rather than burdening the reader with excessive and detailed references and citations in this *Primer*, given below are particularly useful selected references. In addition, other specific references and citations will be given in parentheses throughout the *Primer*. For further information and details about any topics presented and discussed in this book, the interested reader is referred not only to the following list of selected references, but also to applicable textbooks, monographs, electronic databases, print articles and materials, Internet sources, and other applicable resources.

Selected References

Black DW, Andreasen NC. Introductory textbook of psychiatry. 6th ed. American Psychiatric Publishing, Inc.; 2014. (A solid basic textbook of psychiatry.)

Multiple Authors. Diagnostic and statistical manual of mental health disorders (*DSM-5*). 5th ed. American Psychiatry Association, Inc.; 2013. (This book is the controversial "bible" for primarily American and Canadian psychiatric diagnoses.)

The comparable international work to the *DSM-5* is currently the 2019 International classification of diseases (*ICD-10*). 10th ed. World Health Organization. (The *ICD-11* was due for adoption in 2020.)

Frances A. Saving normal: an insider's revolt against out-of-control psychiatric diagnosis, big pharma, and the medicalization of ordinary life. Harper Collins Publishers; 2013. (The subtitle says it all! See Chap. 4 in this *Primer*.)

Ghaemi SN. Clinical psychopharmacology: principles and practice. Oxford University Press; 2019. (A scholarly, detailed, and lengthy overview of psychopharmacology, also covering social practice and research/methodologic aspects of the field.)

Hales RE, Yudofsky ST, Roberts LW, editors, et al. The American Psychiatric Publishing textbook of psychiatry. 6th ed. American Psychiatric Publishing, Inc.; 2014. (A standard, detailed encyclopedic textbook tome, for reference. A seventh edition is available, copyright 2019, with updated coverage in a number of areas.)

Harrington A. Mind fixers: psychiatry's troubled search for the biology of mental illness. W.W. Norton and Company; 2019. (A historical and scholarly review of the topic, including some of the same topics as *Saving Normal* listed above.)

Puzantian T, Carlat DJ. Medication fact book for psychiatric practice. 6th ed. Carlat Publishing, LLC; 2020. (A very useful "cookbook" for psychotropic prescribing, conveniently organized and presented for the practitioner.)

Watters E. Crazy like us: the globalization of the American psyche. Free Press; 2010. (Psychiatric diagnostic issues similar to those in *Saving Normal,* with an international focus.)

Weil A. Mind over meds: know when drugs are necessary, when alternatives are better—and when to let your body heal on its own. Little, Brown and Company; 2017. (A balanced and holistic approach to pharmacology and psychopharmacology by the popular "guru" of these fields.)

Selected Internet References

With the surfeit of internet resources, websites of all imaginable types and quality, and numerous related electronic sources of information and data, the reader, clinician, researcher, and member of the public—patient/client or not—may easily become confused about where to go and what to accept in learning psychopharmacology and psychopharmacotherapy. In this vein, a productive way to navigate the bewildering array of such sources consists of dividing them into several categories, viz.

1. Refereed ("peer-reviewed;" "juried") scientific, technical, and professional journals, newsletters, and the like, including e-journals, e-newsletters, and other open-source e-publications. Selected examples include:

   - *Journal of Clinical Psychopharmacology* (peer-reviewed independent professional journal)
   - *Experimental & Clinical Psychopharmacology* (peer-reviewed professional journal of the American Psychological Association)
   - *Journal of Psychopharmacology* (peer-reviewed professional journal of the British Association for Psychopharmacology)
   - *Psychopharmacology* (Berlin/Heidelberg; Springer Publications)

2. Government and academic/research institutions, publications and e-publications, and associated websites. Selected examples include:

   - National Institute of Mental Health (NIMH) website, affiliated institutes, programs, centers, websites, and publications (electronic and print)
   - National Institute on Alcoholism and Alcohol Abuse (NIAAA) website, affiliated institutes, programs and centers, and websites and publications (electronic and print)
   - National Institute on Drug Abuse (NIDA) website, affiliated institutes, centers, programs and websites, and publications (electronic and print)
   - Canadian Centre on Substance Abuse (CCSA), affiliated programs and publications (electronic and print)
   - National Center on Addiction and Substance Abuse at Columbia University (NCASACU), programs and publications (electronic and print)

3. Journals, magazines, societies, and associated websites. Selected examples include:

   - *Psychology Today*
   - *Scientific American*
   - *Scientific American Mind*

As a practical matter, in researching particular topics electronically in psychopharmacology/psychopharmacotherapy, the logical rule—as with everything else—is to search for topic(s), keyword(s), and the like on a search engine, then to narrow the search with entries given by the search engine. An important factor to keep in mind here is the reliability, accuracy, and quality of the source: Sources from (1) and (2)—above—are considered more reliable than those in (3), generally. Those in (3), in turn, are generally considered more reliable than personal blogs, newsletters, product websites, company websites, and the like.

In the final analysis, the success of this *Primer* will depend on its helpfulness to you, the reader. For that reason, this author welcomes feedback and suggestions to make this book as practical and useful as possible. Please feel free to contact me with suggestions at dpgreenfieldmdpsychiatry@msn.com.

Finally, this book is also *not* intended as a treatment guide for the clinical care of patients/clients. The reader should consult their healthcare professionals/treatment providers for that purpose.

Short Hills, NJ, USA   Daniel P. Greenfield

Acknowledgments

I am particularly grateful to Joann Codella, my dedicated assistant and typist, who worked long, hard, and very well on the manuscript for this book, making this *Primer* possible.

I am also particularly grateful to Joan Van der Veen, my private office manager, whose background and experience in publishing and graphics made her an invaluable asset with the production of this *Primer*.

Many thanks to my friends and colleagues in the Department of Physician Assistant at Seton Hall University, who supported and encouraged this undertaking.

Heartfelt thanks to Christopher J. Hanifin, MS, PA-C, EdD, Chairperson and Program Director of the Department of the Physician Assistant at Seton Hall University, who wrote the Clinical Foreword for this book.

Heartfelt thanks, too, to the Honorable Kevin G. Calahan, JSC (retired) of the Superior Court of New Jersey (Hudson Vicinage) and Professor of Criminal Justice at Saint Peter's University (Jersey City, New Jersey), who wrote the Legal/Forensic Foreword for this book.

Heartfelt thanks, too, to John W. Sensakovic, MD, PhD, a friend and colleague for over thirty years, who first introduced me to Seton Hall University and who has enthusiastically supported and endorsed this book.

Saving the best until last, I acknowledge Alma Scott Greenfield, my oldest grandchild (now 13 years old), for her extraordinary help in organizing the Index for this book. Alma succeeded where others, with many more years and much more experience than she, did not. Alma was a baby when she made her first appearance in the "Dedication" of one of my books. This time, she's been an invaluable part of the publishing process. Thank you, Alma. I couldn't be more proud!

Thank you all very much for your help: I could not have done this *Primer* without you.

Contents

About the Author

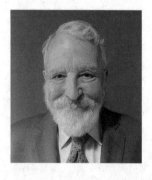

Daniel P. Greenfield, MD, MPH, MS, FASAM is a practicing psychiatrist, addiction medicine specialist, and preventive medicine specialist. He was educated at Oberlin College, the University of North Carolina, the University of London, Cornell University Medical Center, Rutgers University, and Harvard University.

In addition to his clinical and forensic practice, he formerly taught at the Albert Einstein College of Medicine as an attending physician and at Montefiore Medical Center (Bronx, New York) as a Clinical Associate Professor of Psychiatry and Behavioral Science.

He currently teaches at Seton Hall University, where he is a Clinical Professor of Neuroscience (Psychiatry) at the JFK Neuroscience Institute Hackensack Meridian Health/JFK University Medical Center (South Orange, Nutley, and Edison, New Jersey).

He has lectured, published, and testified widely in areas of his background, training, and expertise, in academic, business, community, courtroom, government, and professional forums, as well as on television and radio.

Psychopharmacology for Nonpsychiatrists: A Primer is one of his latest books.

Dr. Greenfield can be reached at dpgreenfieldmdpsychiatry@msn.com.

Chapter 1
Introduction: Epidemiologic Triangle Model, Diagnosis, Psychiatric Diagnosis, and Other Necessary Preliminaries

In a thought-provoking essay entitled "How Prozac Slew Freud," Edward Shorter, historian of science at the University of Toronto, asserted that the psychoanalytic orientation in psychiatry is outmoded and ineffective and that psychopharmacology is the proper orientation and basic skill set for psychiatry. Shorter's opinion is an accurate, if somewhat controversial, depiction of the current state of psychiatry as a branch of medicine. Shorter's assertion highlights the importance of understanding the complexity of psychopharmacology as applied not only in clinical contexts but in forensic and other contexts discussed in this volume, as well. This assertion, in turn, leads to the need to structure psychopharmacology in some way, in order to understand this vast field in comprehensible parts. To start this process, this *Primer* proposes two broad topics leading to proper diagnosis.

The first of these topics is the Epidemiologic Triangle model, consisting of three components, viz., **host**, **environment**, and **agent**. Each component is to be evaluated in the context of its own properties and its interactive effects on the others. A dramatic recent example of this is the COVID-19 epidemic: Specifically, the effect on the host (people) of quarantining and "social distancing" (environment) from the agent (the COVID-19 virus). Medical experts opined that changing the environment earlier in the course of the epidemic to stricter quarantining and social distancing would have considerably reduced the death toll from the epidemic. In psychiatry, for present purposes, we consider the "host" to be the psychiatric patient; the "environment" to be the patient's life circumstances, broadly speaking; and the "agent" to be the psychotropic medication or medications taken by the patient/client.

The second basic topic is "diagnosis." The concept of "diagnosis" (from the Greek "dia-" meaning "thoroughly" or "completely," and "-gnosis" meaning "to know") is an ancient and fundamental cornerstone of medicine. It may be defined as the process of determining by examination the cause and nature of a disease, illness, or condition and is considered essential for proper treatment. Borrowing again from the field of epidemiology, two types of criteria are used to categorize ill persons into groups (i.e., disease entities), namely:

© The Author(s), under exclusive license to Springer Nature Switzerland AG 2022
D. P. Greenfield, *Psychopharmacology for Nonpsychiatrists*, https://doi.org/10.1007/978-3-030-82507-2_1

1. **Manifestational criteria**, in which ill persons are grouped according to similarity with respect to signs, symptoms, changes in body chemistry, physiologic function, and the like. Examples include idiopathic fever of unknown origin (FUO), intellectual disability and—for present purposes—most psychiatric disorders except for those with putative underlying organic causes (Alzheimer's disease; seizure disorders).
2. **Causal criteria**, in which ill persons are grouped according to their similarity with respect to common experience(s) believed to be the cause, or etiology (from the Greek "etios-" meaning "cause," and "-logos" meaning "study of") of their disease, illness, or condition. Examples include coronavirus infections, lead poisoning, and neural tube defect disability. In studying diseases, historical trends have progressed from manifestational (e.g., "pox") to causal (e.g., "syphilis") understanding of a disease.

The concept of "differential diagnosis" in this context is an extension of "diagnosis" and is central to clinical-thinking, reasoning, and problem-solving. "Differential diagnosis" refers to a group, or listing, of potential "causes" of the constellation of signs and symptoms (predominantly manifestational in psychiatric conditions) which best account for the condition or "diagnosis," under consideration. The several potential "causes" of crushing substernal chest pain and shortness of breath—myocardial infarction ("heart attack"), acute respiratory insufficiency from COVID-19 infection, pneumonia, and many others—come to mind as examples from general medicine.

In psychiatric conditions manifesting as acute paranoia, the "differential diagnosis" would include amphetamine overdose, cocaine intoxication, acute psychotic episode, mini-psychotic episode from underlying borderline personality disorder, and others. All of these possibilities need to be "ruled out," or excluded, through appropriate history-taking, testing (including urine drug screen [UDS] or "tox" screen), and other such diagnostic procedures, in order to arrive at a plausible underlying diagnosis and a treatment plan likely to be successful. This is the same model and clinical methodology as with the disciplines of general medicine and surgery.

The third basic concept preliminary to discussing substantive aspects of psychopharmacology and psychopharmacotherapy is "psychiatric diagnosis." This particular system—presently embodied in the Fifth Edition of the *Diagnostic and Statistical Manual of Mental Disorders* (*DSM-5*) of the American Psychiatric Association, copyright 2013—is a hybrid classification system based predominantly on manifestational criteria. With this system, the use of "psychotropic" (from the Greek "psycho-" meaning "soul," and "-tropos" meaning "way" or "manner") medications to ameliorate or control symptomatology due to a putative underlying cause, but not necessarily to address, or "cure," or "eliminate" the cause itself. In that sense, most psychotropic medications act to counter undesirable symptomatology, such as "depression" with "antidepressants," or "psychosis" with "antipsychotics," with varying understandings of the reasons—"mechanism of action" (MOA)—of the underlying disease ("disorder") process. Notwithstanding this limitation, the present iteration of the *Diagnostic and Statistical Manual of Mental Disorders* (*DSM-5*), and its six predecessors—going back to 1952—have been called the "bible" for psychiatric disorders in organized psychiatry.

For present purposes in addressing the need to have a basic understanding of the *DSM-5* for discussing substantive aspects of psychopharmacology/psychopharmacotherapy, the following excerpts from the "Cautionary Statement for Forensic Use of *DSM-5*" (about the inapplicability of adopting the *DSM-5* wholesale for forensic psychiatric purposes) are instructive:

> Although the *DSM-5* diagnostic criteria and text are primarily designed to assist clinicians in conducting clinical assessment, case formulation, and treatment planning, *DSM-5* is also used as a reference for the courts and attorneys in assessing the forensic consequences of mental disorders. As a result, it is important to note that the definition of mental disorder included in *DSM-5* was developed to meet the needs of clinicians, public health professionals, and research investigators rather than all of the technical needs of the courts and legal professionals… the use of *DSM-5* should be informed by an awareness of the risks and limitations of its use in forensic settings… These dangers arise because the imperfect fit between the questions of ultimate concern to the law and the information contained in a clinical diagnosis… [for example]… having the diagnosis in itself does not demonstrate that a particular individual is (or was) unable to control his or her behavior at a particular time… (page 25 of the *DSM-5*)

Put more concisely, in the context of forensic psychiatry (see Part III of this book), the presence of a *DSM-5* **diagnosis** does no more to pinpoint a particular **disability** (level of functioning, or symptomatology, for example) than does the presence of that **diagnosis** to pinpoint a specific **etiology**, causes or mechanism of action, for that diagnosis. This is an important concept in psychopharmacology/psychopharmacotherapy and will be developed and revisited throughout this book.

Recognizing and accepting these limitations and restrictions in psychiatric diagnosis, however, the basis for the several "anti" categories of psychopharmacologic agents in this book (see Part I) will be the *DSM-5*, owing to its widespread acceptability and use in the psychiatric community. In this regard, the reader must be aware of and careful about what one prominent psychiatric insider and commentator has called "diagnostic inflation." This concept refers to increasing apparent prevalence (presence, or frequency), of given psychiatric disorders and conditions based, in part, on *DSM* definitions and diagnostic criteria in successive editions of the *DSM* over the years, regardless of the underlying neurobiological mechanism of action, causes, or etiology of the disorder at issue. This concept is particularly relevant to psychopharmacology/psychopharmacotherapy in terms of the reasons, or clinical indications, for prescribing given agents for particular disorders. If, for example, the apparent prevalence of a psychiatric disorder in a given population increases because of a change—a broadening or widening—in *DSM-5* diagnostic criteria (whether or not that change reflects a true increase in that prevalence), then the prescribing clinician will necessarily prescribe a given psychopharmacologic/psychopharmacotherapeutic agent for more patients or for a broader range of patients with related diagnoses than if the *DSM* diagnostic change had never occurred. This "inflation" has been identified for a number of psychiatric disorders, including attention-deficit hyperactivity disorder (ADHD), eating disorders (anorexia and bulimia), and post-traumatic stress disorder (PTSD), among others.

With all these caveats, Table 1.1 lists the current major categories of psychiatric disorders as given in the *DSM-5*.

In the next part of this book—the core of the book—I will present and discuss substantive and practical aspects of psychopharmacology/psychopharmacotherapy.

Table 1.1 *DSM-5* major diagnostic categories

Neurodevelopmental disorders
Schizophrenia spectrum and other psychotic disorders
Bipolar and related disorders
Depressive disorders
Anxiety disorders
Obsessive-compulsive and related disorders
Trauma and stressor-related disorders
Feeding and eating disorders
Elimination disorders
Sleep-wake disorders
Sexual dysfunction
Gender dysphoria
Disruptive, impulse-control, and conduct disorders
Substance-related and addictive disorders
Neurocognitive disorders
Personality disorders
Paraphilic disorders
Other mental disorders

A Note on References

Rather than burdening the reader with excessive and detailed references and citations in this *Primer*, given below are particularly useful selected references. In addition, other specific references and citations will be given in parentheses throughout the *Primer*. For further information and details about any topics presented and discussed in this book, the interested reader is referred not only to the following list of selected references but also to applicable textbooks, monographs, electronic databases, print articles and materials, internet sources, and other applicable resources.

Selected References

- Black DW, Andreasen NC. Introductory textbook of psychiatry. 6th ed. American Psychiatric Publishing, Inc.; 2014. (A solid basic textbook of psychiatry.)
- Multiple Authors. Diagnostic and statistical manual of mental health disorders (*DSM-5*). 5th ed. American Psychiatry Association, Inc.; 2013. (This book is the controversial "bible" for primarily American and Canadian psychiatric diagnoses.)
- The comparable international work to the *DSM-5* is currently the 2019 International Classification of Diseases (*ICD-10*). 10th ed. World Health Organization. (The *ICD-11* was due for adoption in 2020.)
- Frances A. Saving normal: an insider's revolt against out-of-control psychiatric diagnosis, big pharma, and the medicalization of ordinary life. Harper Collins Publishers: 2013. (The subtitle says it all! See Chap. 4 of this *Primer*.)

- Ghaemi SN. Clinical psychopharmacology: principles and practice. Oxford University Press: 2019. (A scholarly, detailed, and lengthy overview of psychopharmacology, also covering social practice and research/methodologic aspects of the field.)
- Hales RE, Yudofsky ST, Roberts LW, et al., editors. The American Psychiatric Publishing textbook of psychiatry. 6th ed. American Psychiatric Publishing, Inc.; 2014. (A standard, detailed encyclopedic textbook tome, for reference. A seventh edition is available, copyright 2019, with updated coverage in a number of areas.)
- Harrington A. Mind fixers: psychiatry's troubled search for the biology of mental illness. W.W. Norton and Company; 2019. (A historical and scholarly review of the topic, including some of the same topics as *Saving Normal* listed above.)
- Puzantian T, Carlat DJ. Medication fact book for psychiatric practice. 6th ed. Carlat Publishing, LLC; 2020. (A very useful "cookbook" for psychotropic prescribing, conveniently organized and presented for the practitioner.)
- Watters E. Crazy like us: the globalization of the American psyche. Free Press; 2010. (Psychiatric diagnostic issues similar to those in *Saving Normal*, with an international focus.)
- Weil A. Mind over meds: know when drugs are necessary, when alternatives are better—and when to let your body heal on its own. Little, Brown and Company; 2017. (A balanced and holistic approach to pharmacology and psychopharmacology by the popular "guru" of these fields.)

Selected Internet References

With the surfeit of internet resources, websites of all imaginable types and quality, and numerous related electronic sources of information and data, the reader, clinician, researcher, and member of the public—patient/client or not—may easily become confused about where to go and what to accept in learning psychopharmacology and psychopharmacotherapy. In this vein, a productive way to navigate the bewildering array of such sources consists of dividing them into several categories, viz.

1. Refereed ("peer-reviewed;" "juried") scientific, technical, and professional journals, newsletters, and the like, including e-journals, e-newsletters, and other open-source e-publications. Selected examples include:

   - *Journal of Clinical Psychopharmacology* (peer-reviewed independent professional journal)
   - *Experimental & Clinical Psychopharmacology* (peer-reviewed professional journal of the American Psychological Association)
   - *Journal of Psychopharmacology* (peer-reviewed professional journal of the British Association for Psychopharmacology)
   - *Psychopharmacology* (Berlin/Heidelberg; Springer Publications)

2. Government and academic/research institutions, publications and e-publications, and associated websites. Selected examples include:

- National Institute of Mental Health (NIMH) website, affiliated institutes, programs, centers, websites, and publications (electronic and print)
- National Institute on Alcoholism and Alcohol Abuse (NIAAA) website, affiliated institutes, programs and centers, and websites and publications (electronic and print)
- National Institute on Drug Abuse (NIDA) website, affiliated institutes, centers, programs and websites, and publications (electronic and print)
- Canadian Centre on Substance Abuse (CCSA), affiliated programs and publications (electronic and print)
- National Center on Addiction and Substance Abuse at Columbia University (NCASACU), programs and publications (electronic and print)

3. Journals, magazines, societies, and associated websites. Selected examples include:

- *Psychology Today*
- *Scientific American*
- *Scientific American Mind*

As a practical matter, in researching particular topics electronically in psychopharmacology/psychopharmacotherapy, the logical rule—as with everything else—is to search for topic(s), keyword(s), and the like on a search engine, then to narrow the search with entries given by the search engine. An important factor to keep in mind here is the reliability, accuracy, and quality of the source: Sources from (1) and (2)—above—are considered more reliable than those in (3), generally. Those in (3), in turn, are generally considered more reliable than personal blogs, newsletters, product websites, company websites, and the like.

Part I
Essentials of Psychopharmacology and Psychopharmacotherapy

Chapter 2
Basic Principles of Pharmacology, Psychopharmacology, and Psychopharmacotherapy

Concerning concepts and terms in human biology and medicine, the most fundamental life science underlying all of the sciences discussed in this chapter is physiology. The term derives from the Greek "physio-" meaning "nature," and "-logia" meaning "study of." As a basic clinical science, human physiology encompasses the physical and chemical functioning of the normal human organism, unaffected, unchanged, and uninfluenced by disease, licit or illicit substances, "xenobiotics" (foreign substances, from the Greek, "xeno-" meaning "foreign," and "-biota" meaning "living things"), or other such entities.

In contrast, pharmacology (from the Greek, "pharmakon" meaning "drug") refers to the science of the effects on the human organism of foreign substances or agents (i.e., not normally found in the organism or in any of its organ systems or subsystems). Toxicology (from the Greek, "toxikon" meaning "poison") is generally considered a parallel science, or sub science, of pharmacology. Its relationship to pharmacology was captured some 500 years ago in the words of Paracelsus (Philippus Aureolus Theophrastus Bombastus von Hohenheim, a sixteenth-century Swiss physician and natural philosopher who lived from 1493 to 1541), known as the "father of toxicology," who wrote that "…all substances are poisons; there is none which is not a poison. The right dose differentiates a poison from a remedy…" (Klaassen K, et al. Introduction. In Casarett and Doull's toxicology. 4th ed. McGraw-Hill; 1990.)

Finally, psychopharmacology (from the Greek "psyche-" meaning "soul") is the branch of pharmacology which deals with pharmacologic agents, drugs, or medications which act on (psycho**active**) or influence (psycho**tropic**) the mind (or in more current neuroscientific terminology, the brain and nervous system; see above).

Concerning basic principles of pharmacology and psychopharmacology from the perspective of what happens to active psychopharmacologic **agents**, or drugs/medications, when they interact with the human host who is taking them, in any environment in which that individual is taking these agents (i.e., the Epidemiologic Triangle model as discussed in Chap. 1), three concepts are of considerable

© The Author(s), under exclusive license to Springer Nature Switzerland AG 2022
D. P. Greenfield, *Psychopharmacology for Nonpsychiatrists*, https://doi.org/10.1007/978-3-030-82507-2_2

importance. These are (1) dose–response relationships; (2) desired or undesired ("side") effects; and (3) pharmacologic interactions[1]. Each of these will be discussed, in turn, below.

1. **Dose–Response Relationship**

    The concept of the dose–response relationship states that as a pharmacologic agent increases in amount in a host, or organism, the organism's reaction, or response, to that agent increases in a predictable pattern, resulting in one of two characteristic dose–response curves, depending on the nature of the agents and of the host. Generally, this response pattern will demonstrate a greater response to an increased dose, after an initial lag, or induction phase, and will then plateau at the end of the maximal beneficial dose. Graphically, this pattern is demonstrated in an s-shaped or sigmoid dose–response curve, as illustrated in Fig. 2.1.

Another dose–response curve is referred to as a "therapeutic window," in which an initial lag (induction) phase is followed by a rapid increase, then slowing, then plateauing, then a declining response phase, such that an effective range, or "therapeutic window" of response occurs within a low and high dose range of the agent, but not before or after that range. This is illustrated in Fig. 2.1 (below), in which the effective dose range is between the two asterisks on the "Dose" axis of Fig. 2.1.

    The development of **tolerance** to a drug or medication—defined as a state of reduced responsiveness to a drug or medication generally as a result of long-term, repeated exposure to that agent—may alter the dose–response relationship of a person to a particular agent. This phenomenon is particularly characteristic of alcohol and depressant medication, for present purposes.

---

[1] Basic pharmacology distinguishes in this context between **pharmacokinetics** ("What the body does to the drug: absorption, distribution, metabolism, and excretion") and **pharmacodynamics** ("What the drug does to the body: inhibition, facilitation, synergy, or competition between or among drugs at target and receptor sites; drug–drug, drug–food interactions"). In these areas, the hepatic cytochrome oxidase P-450 (CYP) system metabolizes different pharmacologic agents in different ways, requiring the prescriber to know about these ways in terms of drug–drug interactions. Some drugs, for example, operating on certain CYP systems, will competitively accelerate the metabolism of other drugs, making it necessary to prescribe **higher** doses of the affected agent to obtain the desired effect. The opposite can also occur, in which one drug will competitively inhibit the metabolism of other drugs, making it necessary to prescribe **lower** doses of the affected agent to obtain the desired effect. These CYP system relationships are generally well known and well documented (in hard-copy tables and electronically) for psychotropic medications, and the prescriber of prospective psychotropic agents should be aware of these potential drug–drug interactions before prescribing any such medication.

2. Desired and Undesired ("Side") Effects

The concept of desired and undesired ("side") effects, simply stated, asserts that no active pharmacologic or psychopharmacologic agent exhibits only the desired beneficial effects for which it is intended, for a variety of reasons. For example, one such reason, recently understood, asserts that by virtue of their molecular pharmacology, some pharmacologic agents have more than one therapeutic mechanism of action and can be used for different clinical reasons, or indications, in different dose ranges. These agents are called "multifunctional drugs," one widely used example of which is trazadone, an antidepressant (see Chap. 3) with sedating properties.

In any event, all active pharmacologic and psychopharmacology agents will manifest some undesirable ("side") effects to a greater or lesser degree. These side effects may be dose-related (as described in Fig. 2.1) or may be "idiosyncratic" and unpredictable, occurring if a threshold dose of the agent is reached, as in unexpected allergic reactions. In addition, these undesired or side effects may be **specific** (i.e., related to the desired effect of the agent itself, such as excessive sedation from a sedative-hypnotic [sleep-inducing] drug) or **non-specific** (i.e., not related to the desired effect of the pharmacologic agent, such as nausea and diarrhea caused by some antibiotics). The term commonly applied to situations in which an active pharmacologic agent produces an undesired (side effects) response is "adverse drug reactions" (ADR). The current print and/or electronic version of the *Physician's Desk Reference* (*PDR*) and other such electronic databases gives detailed current information about desired and side effects of the medications licensed and approved by the Food and Drug Administration (FDA) in the United States.

Fig. 2.1 Theoretical dose–response curves. (Adapted from Greenfield D. Pharmacology and psychopharmacology. In McDonald JJ, Kulick FB, editors. Mental and emotional injuries in employment litigation, 2nd ed. BNA Books; 2001)

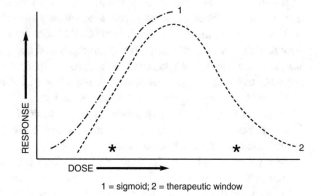

1 = sigmoid; 2 = therapeutic window

3. **Pharmacologic Interactions**

   The third fundamental concept in pharmacology, for present purposes, is pharmacologic interactions. This concept recognizes that once a pharmacologic agent (i.e., drug; medication) is in the body (see footnote 1), chemical interactions with other substances in the body can influence that agent's actions and effectiveness and may require upward or downward changes in doses of that agent (drug/medication) for it to have its desired effects. The most commonly described such interactions are with other drugs (called "drug–drug interactions," or DDIs), with food (called "drug–food interactions" or DFIs), or with underlying medical conditions (such as absorption and metabolic disorders, including malabsorption, diabetes mellitus, and renal insufficiency disorders). The practical implications of these interactions include the potential need for adjustment in doses of a medication in order for it to have its desired and expected response.

   Awareness of these interactions will allow the prescribing practitioner to understand better the potential issues involved in individuals' psychiatric disorders which are being treated by psychotropic medications. In such situations, the variety of factors described in the Epidemiologic Triangle model should be considered, including drug–drug interactions (in the **host**), the living situation of the host (**environment**), the dose–response characteristic of drugs and medications (**agents**), and the interactions of all of these factors.

Classes of Pharmacologic and Psychopharmacologic Agents

For present classification purposes, the initial division of pharmacologic agents will be into **non-psychotropic** and **psychotropic** agents, recognizing that a variety of undesired ("side") effects of a psychiatric, neuropsychiatric, or neurologic nature (e.g., dizziness, fatigue, lethargy, transient sensory disturbances, depression, malaise, and others) may occur with both of these broad classes of pharmacologic agents. The vast majority of both psychotropic and non-psychotropic medications are prescribed by non-psychiatric physicians (primary care physicians, internists, obstetricians-gynecologists, surgeons, orthopedics, and others) and other healthcare providers who may prescribe medications and drugs (e.g., physician assistants, advanced practice nurses, psychologists with prescribing privileges, and others). This is the case simply because there are so many more nonpsychiatrist providers prescribing these agents than there are psychiatrists.

Non-psychotropic medications may be further classified in several ways, including the **organ system** they are intended to affect (e.g., cardiovascular drugs; pulmonary drugs) and the **disease** they are intended to treat (e.g., antineoplastic [anticancer] medications; antidotes for poisoning), with some overlap between the two (e.g., antituberculosis drugs as an example of an anti-infectious agent which primarily affects pulmonary, or lung function, by virtue of the main site of infection of the tuberculosis-causing bacteria). Tables 2.1 and 2.2 give examples of medications/drugs in these two subclasses of non-psychotropic medications.

Examples of side effects of members of both of these classes of non-psychotropic medications are given in Table 2.1.

Table 2.1 Selected examples of non-psychotropic medications classified by the organ system affected

Organ system	Agent (medication)

Cardiovascular	Digitalis preparations (cardiac):
	   Digoxin (various preparations)
	 Antihypertensives:
	   Atenolol (Tenormin®)
	   Alphamethyldopa (Aldomet®)
	   Beta-propranolol (Inderal®)

Gastrointestinal	Motility agents:
	   Metoclopramide (Reglan®)
	 Antacids:
	   Maalox®
	   Mylanta®
	 Histamine blockers:
	   Cimetidine (Tagamet®)
	   Ranitidine (Zantac®)

Endocrine/ metabolic	Diabetes mellitus preparations:
	   Humulin®
	   NPH
	   Oral hypoglycemic
	 Thyroid replacement preparations:
	   Cytomel®
	   Synthroid®

Pulmonary	Bronchodilators:
	   Isoproterenol (Isuprel®)
	   Epinephrine

Integumentary (skin)	Topical steroids:
	   Retin-A®
	   Cortisone®

Table 2.2 Selected examples of non-psychotropic medications classified by diseases treated

Disease	Agent (medication)

Infectious diseases (pneumonia, meningitis, AIDS)	Antibiotics and antivirals:
	   Penicillin
	   Cephaloxin (Keflex®)
	   Erythromycin
	   Zidovudine (Retrovir®)

Neoplastic diseases (cancers)	Methotrexate Steroids Aspirin Nonsteroidal anti-inflammatory drugs (NSAIDs)
Immunological diseases	Steroids Azulfidine Imuran®
Degenerative central nervous system (CNS) diseases	L-Dopa, Sinemet® (for Parkinson's disease)

Poisoning	Syrup of ipecac
	 Chelating agents:
	   EDTA
	   Penicillamine

Psychotropic Medications, for purposes of the "anti" classification system presented in this book, may be further divided in several ways, with overlap among members of these divisions. These divisions are (1) **Licit** and **Illicit** drugs and medications (so designated according to the lawfulness of their use. **Stimulants**, **depressants**, and **hallucinogens** are medications/drugs in this class) and (2) twenty categories of medications and drugs, for present purposes (so designated according to the predominant clinical indication, or reason, or condition/psychiatric disorder treated with the medication, recognizing that many of these are indicated—FDA-approved or off-label[2]—for treatment of more than one condition or illness), as presented and discussed in further detail in Chaps. 3 and 4 of this volume. Table 2.3 illustrates these two classification systems of psychotropic drugs/medications.

Table 2.3 Licit and illicit psychotropic agents

Licit psychotropic Drugs/medications	Illicit psychotropic Drugs/medications
"Twenty Anti-s" (see Table 2.5 below; see Chaps. 3 and 4)	**Stimulants, depressants, hallucinogens** (see Chap. 5)

---

[2] "Approval by the Food and Drug Administration (FDA) implies that available evidence shows that a drug is safe and effective for the specific indication (disease or symptom) for which it is tested…" whereas the term off-label as currently used "…commonly refers to prescribing currently available medication for an indication (disease or symptom) for which it has not received FDA approval…[that it is] not the same as experimental or research use… Once a drug is FDA-approved for a specific indication, legally it can be used for any indication…" (Furey K, Wilkins K. AMA Journal of Ethics, 2016). As will be discussed later in this *Primer*, many available psychotropic agents are frequently prescribed off-label today. Practically speaking, these prescribing patterns are so much the case, for example, that there is a specific section for each of the entries for specific psychotropic medications in Puzantian and Carlat's Medication Fact Book (see Selected References, in the Preface of this book) is for "off-label uses."

1. **Classification according to Lawfulness of Use (Licit and Illicit Psychotropic Agents)**

   "Licit" agents are those that may be prescribed and taken legally (such as prescription medications and over-the-counter [OTC] medications, which may be obtained without a prescription), and "Illicit" agents are those that may not. The latter are typically drugs of abuse, or "street drugs," although areas of overlap are often seen between these two categories. One such example is diversion (from a prescription) to the street of alprazolam (Xanax®), a widely used anti-panic and antianxiety medication (see Chaps. 3 and 4). Another example is the street use of illicitly manufactured psychostimulants, such as methamphetamines ("crystal meth"), a widely used psychostimulant drug of abuse with a wide range of devastating medical and psychiatric consequences. Chapter 5 in this book discusses examples of illicit substances in further detail.

2. **Classification according to the Predominant Psychoactive Effect**

   Psychotropic agents generally produce one of three psychoactive effects in their users, viz., **stimulation** (excitement, agitation, acceleration of thought and speech, and otherwise "speeding up" of the user); **depression** (dulling, deceleration of thought and speech, and otherwise "slowing down" of the user); and **psychosis** (a break with reality, having hallucinations, and/or having delusional thoughts. "Hallucinogens" which caused these symptoms, such as PCP, are also known as "psychomimetics" or "mimicking psychosis"). Table 2.4 gives representative examples of drugs (illicit) and medications in these three classes.

Table 2.4 Examples of illicit (and divertible; see Chap. 5) psychotropic agents

Stimulants
Amphetamines and related compounds (sympathomimetics)
Cocaine
Depressants
Alcohol (ethanol)
Heroin and other opioids
Sedative-hypnotics
Anxiolytics
Hallucinogens ("psychotomimetic")
Inhalants (especially nitrates)
Lysergic acid diethylamide (LSD)
Marijuana (cannabinol and related compounds)
MDMA ("ecstasy") and other "designer drugs"
Phencyclidine (PCP)
Psilocybin

3. **Classification according to Predominant Clinical Indication Or Reason for Prescribing**

As briefly noted in Table 2.3, members of this group of "licit" drugs and medications may be divided into 20 classes, according to the predominant clinical condition or disorder treated. They are designated with an "anti" prefix to convey their use in "combating" manifestational symptomatology of the intended disorder to treat, regardless of the potential underlying cause, or mechanism, symptoms of the disorder. As with any drug or medication, they can be abused or diverted from legitimate use. But their inclusion in the "licit" category of psychotropic agents, for present purposes, is intended to emphasize that when legitimately used as directed, these drugs and medications have bona fide and legal clinical indications. Chapter 3 ("The Four 'Major Anti-s'") of this book discusses the four most widely used classes of psychotropic medications. Chapter 4 ("The Sixteen 'Minor Anti-s'") discusses the 16 less widely used classes of psychotropic medications, especially by psychiatrists and other mental health practitioners (Table 2.5).

Table 2.5 Licit psychotropic agents: the "twenty anti-s"

Anti-addiction agents
Anti-aggression agents
Antianxiety agents (anxiolytics; minor tranquilizers)
Anti-appetite agents (anorexiants)
Anticonvulsant agents (antiseizure agents; antiepileptic drugs [AEDs])
Anti-dementia agents (cognition enhancers)
Antidepression agents (mood elevators; thymoleptics)
Anti-feeding and eating agents
Anti-hyperactivity agents (psychostimulants)
Anti-impotence agents
Anti-insomnia agents (sedative-hypnotics)
Antimanic agents (mood stabilizers and thymoleptics)
Anti-obsessive-compulsive disorders (OCD) agents
Antipain agents (analgesics)
Antipanic agents
Antiparkinsonian agents
Antipseudobulbar affect agents
Antipsychotic agents (neuroleptics; major tranquilizers)
Antisex agents
Antitrauma agents

Three Additional Classes

Three heterogeneous types of drugs and medications whose members are frequently encountered in clinical and legal/forensic practice which have considerable overlap with the more discrete and unitary 20 subclasses of "Anti-Agent" medications discussed above and in Chaps. 3, 4, and 5 of this book are "Over-the-Counter (OTC) Agents;" "Anticholinergic Agents;" and "Botanicals, Herbals, Nutraceuticals, and (Dietary) Supplements" (BHNSs). These agents do not "fit" conveniently into the other categories or classes presented in this book, and will therefore be discussed as separate categories.

1. **Over-the-Counter (OTC) Drugs and Medications**
   Over-the-Counter (OTC) drugs and medications are a heterogeneous collection of wide-ranging agents, many of which have psychoactive properties, and some of which are marketed as psychotropic medications. The only feature common to these agents, for present classification purposes, is that they are available without prescription, and in that sense—for present purposes—may be considered as comparable to botanicals, herbals, nutraceuticals, and (dietary) supplements (BHNSs; see Chap. 6). The regulation of OTC preparations by the Federal Food and Drug Administration (FDA) periodically permits what the National Pharmaceutical Manufacturers Association calls a "prescription-to-OTC switch," which is generally of considerable financial advantage to the pharmaceutical company that manufactures the switched medication. Bases for such switches include a switch of the medication itself with respect to OTC status and switch approval of a reduced dose level of a medication (such as cimetidine, or Tagamet®, for treatment of gastric hyperacidity). Since these switches may occur with medications which have psychoactive effects and DDIs and DFIs with both psychoactive and non-psychoactive undesired ("side") effects, it behooves prescribers, and anybody else evaluating medical and clinical records (e.g., forensic experts) to be aware of the potentially confounding symptomatic effects OTC medications and drugs may have on patients. Put more simply, when possible, a drug and medication history should always be taken from the evaluee, including both prescribed and OTC medications.

2. **Anticholinergic Drugs and Medications**
   In terms of the anatomy and physiology of the human nervous system,[3] like all nerve cells in the nervous system generally, those of the parasympathetic

---

[3] Very briefly, the human nervous system may be classified into two pairs of dichotomous categories. Anatomically, the nervous system consists of the **central nervous system**, or "CNS" (the brain and spinal cord) and the **peripheral nervous system**, or "PNS" (all other parts of the nervous system outside the brain and spinal cord). Physiologically, and functionally, the nervous system consists of the **voluntary nervous system** and the **involuntary**, or **autonomic nervous system** (ANS). The voluntary nervous system mediates and coordinates involuntary human activities such as digestion, salivation, heart activity, and many others. In many body functions—such as breathing—voluntary and involuntary components exist and overlap and are mediated and coordinated with both voluntary and involuntary input. Anatomically, the ANS consists of two subsystems, the

("slowing down" involuntary bodily functions, such as salivation, digestion, and so forth) division of the autonomic nervous system (ANS) communicate from one to another across a very small space that separates them (the "synapse") with different chemical substances called "neurotransmitters." The predominant neurotransmitter in the parasympathetic nervous system is acetylcholine, and the functions of the parasympathetic nervous system which are mediated by this neurotransmitter are called "cholinergic." Medications, drugs, and other substances which interrupt, disrupt, or otherwise block the cholinergic-mediated functions are called "anticholinergic." A wide variety of substances, medications, drugs, and other chemicals have anticholinergic properties, and in that sense, these substances constitute a heterogeneous group of entities which do not have a single, unitary, or underlying pattern of clinical indications.

That varied group of substances may affect (as undesired, or "side" effects) many of the drugs and medications in the classes of psychotropic drugs discussed in this part of this book: For that reason, psychotropic drugs and medications which block, or disrupt parasympathetic/cholinergic functioning of the ANS, again, are said to have "anticholinergic side effects."

"Somatic" (related to the **body**, in contrast to "psychic" related to the mind) anticholinergic side effects commonly seen with anticholinergic drugs and medications include dry mouth, blurry vision, constipation, urinary hesitancy, and tachycardia (rapid heart rate). Central nervous system ("psychic" or "psychiatric/neuropsychiatric/anticholinergic") signs and symptoms may include organic brain symptomatology (memory impairment, disorientation, confusion, and delirium, among others). The often-heard clinical aphorism which summarizes both the somatic (peripheral) and psychic (central) symptomatology of the anticholinergic syndrome is: "**Red** as a beet; **dry** as a bone; **hot** as hell; and **mad** as a hatter." Examples of medications with anticholinergic effects and side effects include many of the anti-Parkinson's agents (see Chap. 4), antispasmodic gastrointestinal and genitourinary medications, and medications for treating glaucoma (see above).

For legal professionals reading this book in the context of litigation, the feelings of discomfort, dysphoria, and irritability resulting from the anticholinergic syndrome for legitimately prescribed drugs and medications may be incorrectly attributed to events and experiences in the context of the litigation (i.e., rather than to the condition for which the medications are prescribed), and/or to the anticholinergic side effects of the medications themselves. As with all legal cases involving any drugs or medications, the law practitioner and expert should be

---

sympathetic nervous system (SNS)—which speeds up involuntary body activities—and the parasympathetic nervous system—which slows down involuntary body activities. The central portion of the ANS is found in two chains of nerve collections, or "ganglia," located parallel to and on either side of the spinal cord and vertebral column, and in the other ganglia and peripheral nerves located throughout the body. The central part of the ANS is located within the brain and spinal cord.

aware of the litigant's drug and medication history (licit and illicit), if applicable, as well as the litigant's present drug and medication use, if applicable.

3. **Botanicals, Herbals, Nutraceuticals, and (Dietary) Supplements**

The last category of psychopharmacologic agents and substances discussed in this book is also a broad one, and also encompasses overlap among subcategories. This category consists of Botanicals, Herbals, Nutraceuticals, and "Dietary" Supplements (BHNSs), which are reviewed in greater detail in Chap. 6. Several common features characterize this group of four types of substances. **All** are considered "natural" and many are plant-based; **none** is regulated by the FDA as drugs and medications in this country; and **none** is represented to the public as a medication or pharmacologic treatment for a medical condition. Definitions of each of these four members of this varied category of substances are:

- **Botanicals** are plant products, or derived from plants, and are available without prescription from supermarkets, health food and nutrition stores, pharmacies and drug stores, catalogs and internet sources, and other commercial sources.
- **Herbals**—a term to be contrasted with that of a book containing the names and descriptions of plants, usually with information on their properties— refers to plants and plant extracts used by consumers and practitioners in health care in the fields of "botanical medicine," "medical herbalism," "herbal medicine," "herbology," and "phytotherapy."
- **Nutraceuticals,** or **Nutriceuticals**, are, according to *Webster's College Dictionary* (*Webster's College Dictionary*, 2000), "…food[s] or natural substance[s] that contain or [are] supplemented with ingredients purported to have health benefits." The word itself is a condensation of "nutrition" and "pharmaceutical" (from the Latin, "druggist," originally "poisoner"), intended to convey the therapeutic value of such compounds.
- **(Dietary) Supplements**, also called "food supplements" and "nutritional supplements," are preparations which are intended to supplement an individual's diet. These supplements consist of vitamins, minerals, herbs, or other botanicals (excluding tobacco and tobacco products), amino acids, fatty acids, fiber, or other nutrients that are not consumed in sufficient quantity in the diet (DHEA, pregnenolone [a steroid hormone], and the pineal hormone melatonin are marketed as dietary supplements in the United States).

For both clinical and legal practitioners, for present purposes, similar feelings of discomfort, dysphoria, anxiety, irritability, depression, and other such symptomatology may also result from the use of BHNSs in a variety of circumstances, even though public perception of these substances is that they are beneficial and benign (Blendon R, et al. Annals of internal medicine. American College of Physicians; 2001). For that reason, as with all situations involving drugs and/or medications, the practitioner should be aware of patients' (or litigants,' for the legal professional) BHNS history and current use, if applicable, as well as of the patient's or litigant's drug and medication history and current use (licit and illicit), if applicable. As with drugs and medications, a thorough history of the patient's or litigant's BHNS use and history are basic requirements for any clinical or legal professional in this area.

Two Additional Concepts (For All Pharmacologic Agents)

The following two aphorisms apply to two important concepts for all pharmacologic agents, respectively, viz.:

Drugs don't work in patients who don't take them…
— C. Everett Koop, MD, Former U.S. Surgeon General (1982–1989)

The Powerful Placebo
— Title of *JAMA (Journal of the American Medical Association)* article in 1955 by H. K. Beecher

These concepts—compliance/adherence and placebo/nocebo, respectively—to which these aphorisms are valid for all pharmacologic agents, and for psychopharmacotherapeutic medications in particular, given the often-subjective nature of psychiatric and neuropsychiatric symptomatology. Each will be discussed, in turn, below.

1. **Compliance/Adherence**
    The term, "compliance," dates back to 1976 and refers to the extent to which patients obey ("comply with") healthcare providers' instructions about medications, appointments, diet, exercise, and the like. In 2003, recognizing the authoritarian and paternal connotations of the term "compliance," the World Health Organization introduced the term "adherence" as a substitute, to convey the notion of patients' collaboration with providers in their mutual efforts for patients to "adhere" ("stick to") a previously worked out and agreed upon treatment plan (including medications).
    Whatever term is used, compliance/adherence with treatment plans has been problematic in healthcare "since forever," and "…between thirty and 50% of medicines for long-term conditions are not taken as prescribed…[and]…rates of non-adherence in patients with psychotic disorders are comparable to those of patients with other long-term conditions…" (Chapman S, Horne R. Medication nonadherence and psychiatry. In Current opinion in psychiatry. 2020, September. https://journals.lww.com/co-psychiatry/Fulltext/2013/09000/Medication_nonadherence_and_psychiatry.5.aspx).
    A number of approaches for enhancing compliance/adherence among patients has been suggested, including patient education (focusing on the reasons for medications and anticipating and coping with side effects); pill counts, new technologies (e.g., "smart pills," electronically monitored); simplified dosing schedules; patient aids (such as weekly pill boxes); and others.
    Although a detailed discussion of compliance/adherence is beyond the scope of this chapter, for practical purposes, if a prescription for a psychotropic agent does not seem to be producing desired results, the **first** possibility to occur to the

healthcare provider should be that their patient is not taking the medication as prescribed, or at all. Other possibilities include an improper dose, insufficient duration of the medication, drug–drug or drug–food interactions with the medication, treating the patient for an incorrect diagnosis for the prescribed medications, or some combination of all of these possibilities.

2. **Placebo/Nocebo**

Given the subjective and "anti-manifestational" nature of the symptomatology to be addressed by psychopharmacologic agents, no discussion of them would be complete without some attention to "placebos" (from the Latin: "I will please") and "nocebos" (from the Latin: "I will harm"). Both terms refer to effects—desirable and undesirable, respectively—attributed to otherwise inert and inactive substances which were not anticipated or expected. Placebos have been recognized for many years, used in general medicine (sometimes with questionable ethics, which will not be further discussed here) for some 200 years, and recognized specifically in psychiatry for about 60 years. The use of placebo methodology in pharmacologic study design as an indication of negative activity (i.e., in comparison with the active drug, or agent, under study) has also been the standard approach to such studies for many years, although recent findings have documented neurophysiologic activity producing specific neuropsychiatric effects in an otherwise presumably "inert" agent. (Weimer K, Colloca L, Enck Prof. P. Placebo effects in psychology: mediators and moderators. In Lancet psychiatry. 2015, March. https://www.thelancet.com/journals/lanpsy/article/PIIS2215-0366(14)00092-3/fulltext).

"Placebos" and "Nocebos" in the context of psychiatry and psychopharmacology will each be discussed, in turn, below.

Concerning **placebos** in psychiatry and psychopharmacotherapy, with subjective symptomatology such as pain, anxiety, and depression, the role of the "placebo effect" and in that sense, a positive expectation of symptom relief, must always be taken into account in the clinical assessment of a patient's response to a trial of a new medication or treatment intervention. If a patient does not experience expected and anticipated symptom relief, then compliance/adherence, or other issues (see above) may be at play, or the patient may harbor a surreptitious or unknown negative attitude (nocebo effect; see below) toward the intervention.

Concerning **nocebos** in psychiatry and psychopharmacotherapy, perhaps the most practical way to characterize the negative expectations of patients for whom a medication may prove to have a "nocebo effect" can be appreciated in the old saw often heard from patients: "I don't want to be on any medication. I don't even take an aspirin when I have a headache…" While this saw may be a prevalent sentiment among patients, an actual nocebo effect from a specific medication needs to be carefully evaluated on an individual basis, as a practical matter, as part of the differential diagnosis for such unsuccessful medications.

As with considerations of compliance/adherence, a detailed discussion of placebos and nocebos is beyond the scope of this *Primer*. For further information and details about fascinating, evolving, and widespread phenomena, the reader is referred to the many technical and encyclopedic textbooks, articles, monographs, and references available in psychopharmacology and pharmacology.

COVID-19, Telemedicine, Telepsychiatry, and Psychopharmacology

Telemedicine and telepsychiatry are here to stay, even before the COVID-19 pandemic, and especially since the pandemic began. Recognition of the advantages of this means of patient care, especially in underserved settings (e.g., rural, correctional, emergency departments, dense urban areas, and the like), has resulted in the near doubling of telepsychiatry services in the U.S. mental health facilities from 2010 to 2017 (Frank B, Peterson T, Gupta S, Peterson T. Telepsychiatry: what you need to know. In Current psychiatry. 2020, June. https://www.mdedge.com/psychiatry/article/222686/coronavirus-updates/telepsychiatry-what-you-need-know). Concerning psychopharmacotherapy, the relaxation, both formally and informally, of some requirements for mental health patient care owing to the exigencies of the COVID pandemic has led to modification, in this writer's view, of one of the "sacred cows" of prescribing, namely face-to-face examination (including physical examination) of prospective patients for whom psychopharmacotherapy may be considered as part of their treatment plan.

Without purporting to offer the final word in a changing practice environment with multiple moving parts, I echo the **caveat** given in the above article in *Current Psychiatry* concerning medicolegal aspects of telemedicine, telepsychiatry, and even forensic (consulting and correctional)[4] telepsychiatry.

> …When conducting telepsychiatry services, clinicians need to consider several legal issues, including federal and state regulations, as well as professional liability…[and that]…Because state laws related to telepsychiatry are continuously evolving we suggest that clinicians continually check these laws and obtain a regulatory response in writing so there is ongoing documentation… (Joshi KG. Telepsychiatry during COVID-19: understanding the rules. In Current psychiatry. 2020, June. https://www.mdedge.com/psychiatry/article/222695/coronavirus-updates/telepsychiatry-during-covid-19-understanding-rules)

Since the varied, changing, and complex nature of telemedicine, telepsychiatry, and "telepsychopharmacotherapy" is well beyond the scope of this brief section—before, during, and after the COVID-19 pandemic—the reader is referred to the burgeoning literature on this topic, several of which have been referenced in this book.

---

[4] For present purposes, "consultation" forensic psychiatry in contrast to "therapeutic" forensic psychiatry refers to the application of principles of clinical psychiatry and human behavior in criminal, civil, and family areas of the law. "Therapeutic" psychiatry refers to clinical treatment of individuals in civilian settings (mental health centers, hospitals, and so forth); or in custodial settings (jails, prisons, federal penitentiaries, and the like, also known as "correctional psychiatry" (in the United States) and "prison psychiatry" (in the United Kingdom).

A Note on References

Rather than burdening the reader with excessive and detailed references and citations in this *Primer*, given below are particularly useful selected references. In addition, other specific references and citations will be given in parentheses throughout the *Primer*. For further information and details about any topics presented and discussed in this book, the interested reader is referred not only to the following list of selected references but also to applicable textbooks, monographs, electronic databases, print articles and materials, internet sources, and other applicable resources.

Selected References

- Black DW, Andreasen NC. Introductory textbook of psychiatry. 6th ed. American Psychiatric Publishing, Inc.; 2014. (A solid basic textbook of psychiatry.)
- Multiple Authors. Diagnostic and statistical manual of mental health disorders (*DSM-5*). 5th ed. American Psychiatry Association, Inc.; 2013. (This book is the controversial "bible" for primarily American and Canadian psychiatric diagnoses.)
- The comparable international work to the *DSM-5* is currently the 2019 International Classification of Diseases (*ICD-10*). 10th ed. World Health Organization. (The *ICD-11* was due for adoption in 2020.)
- Frances A. Saving normal: an insider's revolt against out-of-control psychiatric diagnosis, big pharma, and the medicalization of ordinary life. Harper Collins Publishers: 2013. (The subtitle says it all! See Chap. 4 in this *Primer*.)
- Ghaemi SN. Clinical psychopharmacology: principles and practice. Oxford University Press: 2019. (A scholarly, detailed, and lengthy overview of psychopharmacology, also covering social practice and research/methodologic aspects of the field.)
- Hales RE, Yudofsky ST, Roberts LW, et al., editors. The American Psychiatric Publishing textbook of psychiatry. 6th ed. American Psychiatric Publishing, Inc.; 2014. (A standard, detailed encyclopedic textbook tome, for reference. A seventh edition is available, copyright 2019, with updated coverage in a number of areas.)
- Harrington A. Mind fixers: psychiatry's troubled search for the biology of mental illness. W.W. Norton and Company; 2019. (A historical and scholarly review of the topic, including some of the same topics as *Saving Normal* listed above.)
- Puzantian T, Carlat DJ. Medication fact book for psychiatric practice. 6th ed. Carlat Publishing, LLC; 2020. (A very useful "cookbook" for psychotropic prescribing, conveniently organized and presented for the practitioner.)
- Watters E. Crazy like us: the globalization of the American psyche. Free Press; 2010. (Psychiatric diagnostic issues similar to those in *Saving Normal*, with an international focus.)

- Weil A. Mind over meds: know when drugs are necessary, when alternatives are better—and when to let your body heal on its own. Little, Brown and Company; 2017. (A balanced and holistic approach to pharmacology and psychopharmacology by the popular "guru" of these fields.)

Selected Internet References

With the surfeit of internet resources, websites of all imaginable types and quality, and numerous related electronic sources of information and data, the reader, clinician, researcher, and member of the public—patient/client or not—may easily become confused about where to go and what to accept in learning psychopharmacology and psychopharmacotherapy. In this vein, a productive way to navigate the bewildering array of such sources consists of dividing them into several categories, viz.

1. Refereed ("peer-reviewed;" "juried") scientific, technical, and professional journals, newsletters, and the like, including e-journals, e-newsletters, and other open-source e-publications. Selected examples include:

   - *Journal of Clinical Psychopharmacology* (peer-reviewed independent professional journal)
   - *Experimental & Clinical Psychopharmacology* (peer-reviewed professional journal of the American Psychological Association)
   - *Journal of Psychopharmacology* (peer-reviewed professional journal of the British Association for Psychopharmacology)
   - *Psychopharmacology* (Berlin/Heidelberg; Springer Publications)

2. Government and academic/research institutions, publications and e-publications and associated websites. Selected examples include:

   - National Institute of Mental Health (NIMH) website, affiliated institutes, programs, centers, websites, and publications (electronic and print)
   - National Institute on Alcoholism and Alcohol Abuse (NIAAA) website, affiliated institutes, programs and centers, and websites and publications (electronic and print)
   - National Institute on Drug Abuse (NIDA) website, affiliated institutes, centers, programs and websites, and publications (electronic and print)
   - Canadian Centre on Substance Abuse (CCSA), affiliated programs and publications (electronic and print)
   - National Center on Addiction and Substance Abuse at Columbia University (NCASACU), programs and publications (electronic and print)

3. Journals, magazines, societies, and associated websites. Selected examples include:

   - *Psychology Today*

- *Scientific American*
- *Scientific American Mind*

As a practical matter, in researching particular topics electronically in psycho-pharmacology/psychopharmacotherapy, the logical rule—as with everything else—is to search for topic(s), keyword(s), and the like on a search engine, then to narrow the search with entries given by the search engine. An important factor to keep in mind here is the reliability, accuracy, and quality of the source: Sources from (1) and (2)—above—are considered more reliable than those in (3), generally. Those in (3), in turn, are generally considered more reliable than personal blogs, newsletters, product websites, company websites, and the like.

Chapter 3
The Four "Major Anti-s"

In Part I of this book—the core of this *Primer*—the substance of psychopharmaco-therapeutic agents used for the treatment and management of psychiatric disorders will be presented, reviewed, and discussed. This review begins in this chapter with the most common, or prevalent, psychiatric disorders seen in clinical practice. These disorders are presented in Table 3.1, along with the designation used in this book of the "anti"-psychotropic medication indicated for treatment and management of these disorders.

Table 3.1 Prevalent psychiatric disorders and their "anti" psychopharmacotherapeutic agents: the four "major anti-s"

Psychiatric disorders	"Anti" psychopharmacotherapeutic agents
Anxiety disorders	"Antianxiety agents"
Depressive disorders	"Antidepressant agents"
Mood instability disorders	"Antimanic agents"
Psychotic disorders	"Antipsychotic agents"

D. P. Greenfield, *Psychopharmacology for Nonpsychiatrists*, https://doi.org/10.1007/978-3-030-82507-2_3

Antianxiety Agents

The first of the four most common psychiatric disorders and their psychopharmaco-therapeutic treatment are "anxiety disorders."

In Chap. 2 of this book, reference was made to the *DSM-5* as an organizing principle for the 20 "anti" categories of psychotropic medications endorsed in this *Primer*. Reference was also made to the *DSM-5* as an imperfect document, not truly "carving nature at her joints" (à la Plato) with respect to mental illness diagnoses. This latter point had been made earlier in a landmark *New York Times* article on January 18, 2015 on "Redefining Mental Illness" by T.R. Luhrmann, as follows:

> ...For decades, American psychiatric science took diagnosis to be fundamental. These categories—depression, schizophrenia, post-traumatic stress disorder—were assumed to represent biologically distinct diseases, and the goal of the research was to figure out the biology of the disease. That didn't pan out. In 2013, the Institute's [National Institute of Mental Health] director, Thomas R. Insel, announced that psychiatric science had failed to find unique biological mechanisms associated with specific diagnoses. What genetic underpinnings or neural circuits they had identified were mostly common across diagnostic groups...
>
> ...And so the Institute has begun one of the most interesting and radical experiments in scientific research in years... Under a program called Research Domain Criteria, all research must begin from a matrix of neuroscientific structures (genre, calls, circuits) that cut across behavioral, cognitive, and social domains (acute fear, loss, arousal). To use an example from the program's website, psychiatric researchers will no longer study people with anxiety; they will study fear circuitry...

For present purposes in this book, however, psychiatric research has not reached the point of having psychopharmacology geared toward ameliorating or resolving a dysfunctional "matrix of neuroscientific structures" which were not "common across diagnostic groups." For now, prescribers of psychotropic medications must settle for the admittedly sloppy and imprecise mélange of overlapping manifestational (i.e., not causal, or etiologic; see Chap. 1) clusters of symptomatology on which the *DSM-5* is based. As pointed out earlier, most currently used psychotropic medications are intended to counter, reduce, ameliorate, or be "anti" to symptomatology resulting from designated disorders. Hence, the 20 "anti" categories of psychotropic medications is the classification system that is used in this book.

Starting with what have been called the "common colds" of psychiatry—"Anxiety" and "Depression," often with overlapping symptomatology common to both—Table 3.2 presents psychotropic medications commonly used as "anxiolytics," "sedative-hypnotics," or "antianxiety drugs," or (in older terminology) "minor tranquilizers."[1] Note that by virtue of overlapping symptomatology treated by different classes of psychotropic medications, several types of psychotropic medications may be used for the same clinical indication[2] (e.g., SSRI antidepressants for anxiety relief).

---

[1] So-called in the 1960s and 1970s to contrast these agents with "major tranquilizers" or antipsychotic medications, used to treat "major" psychoses, not "minor" neuroses. Note that the word, or concept, of "neurosis" is not endorsed as a level of symptomatology or as a diagnostic category and does not appear in the *DSM-5*.

[2] Often "off-label," or not as a formal recognized and approved clinical indication by the Food and Drug Administration (FDA). A substantial proportion of psychotropic medications are prescribed in this way, by both nonpsychiatrists and psychiatrists. (See Chap. 2.)

Table 3.2 Anxiolytic/sedative (daytime)-hypnotic (nighttime) agents

Generic name[*]	Brand name[*]
Benzodiazepines (BDZs) used as daytime anxiolytics	
Alprazolam	Xanax®; XanaxER®
Alprazolam extended release	XanaxER® Librium®
Chlordiazepoxide	Klonopin®
Clonazepam	Tranxene®
Clorazepate	Valium®
Diazepam	Ativan®
Lorazepam	Serax®
Oxazepam	
Nonbenzodiazepines used as daytime anxiolytics	
Buspirone	Buspar®
Benzodiazepines used as nighttime hypnotics (GABAergic agonists)	
Estazolam	Prosom®
Flurazepam	Dalmane®
Quazepam	Doral®
Temazepam	Restoril®
Triazolam	Halcion®
Nonbenzodiazepines used as nighttime hypnotics (GABA-BDZ receptor agonists)	
Eszopiclone	Lunesta®
Zaleplon	Sonata®
Zolpidem	Ambien®
Zolpidem extended release	AmbienCR®
Ramelteon	Rozerem® (melatonin agonist)
Nonbenzodiazepines with anxiolytic/sedating effects (antihistamines)	
Diphenhydramine	Benadryl® (others[a])
Doxepin	Sinequan® (at low doses; antipsychotic at high doses)
Hydroxyzine	Atarax®; Vistaril®
Quetiapine	Seroquel® (at low doses; antipsychotic at high doses)
Nonbenzodiazepines with anxiolytic/sedating effects (adrenergic receptor blocking agents)	
Propranolol	Inderal®
Clonidine	Catapres®

[*]With off-patient medications, different pharmaceutical companies may manufacture the same psychotropic agent, resulting in different brand names for the same "generic equivalent"

Without reiterating details of types and subtypes of *DSM-5* classifications of anxiety disorders—to which the reader is referred for further information and details—the following two case vignettes (one, an old joke, and the other an actual brief case vignette) illustrate psychopharmacotherapeutic approaches to individuals with generalized anxiety disorder (GAD) and panic disorder, respectively. The reader is referred to previously mentioned sources and references for such details and information as dosing schedules, doses, desired and side effects, indications and contraindications, and the like.

A 38-year-old woman from the suburbs consulted her primary care physician assistant (PA) with complaints of severe tension and anxiety, insomnia, overeating, stage fright, and a pervasive sense of dread and foreboding. After interviewing and examining the patient, the PA determined that there was no obvious pathophysiologic basis for the patient's anxiety and prescribed a sedating benzodiazepine estazolam (Prosom®) for her. He instructed her to keep a daily mood diary, to call the practice or follow-up a week before the next scheduled appointment, and to return for a follow-up visit in two weeks. The patient returned as scheduled, appearing calmer, well-rested, energetic, and with a 5-pound weight loss. She told the PA "Ever since I started giving the medication to my husband, I've felt 1000% better. Thank you so much!"

AB, a 48-year-old prominent local academic psychiatric APN has had a longstanding history of stress-related panic disorder (see Chap. 4, also) which had begun abruptly (i.e., her first "herald attacks") in her 30s. Her attacks were associated with public speaking at academic events (conferences, symposia, meetings, and the like). At first, she accepted psychopharmacotherapy alone ("monotherapy") with alprazolam (Xanax®) but became dependent on it after a few months. She then began a course of exercise and cognitive behavioral therapy (CBT), supplemented with paroxetine (Paxil®), which had recently received FDA approval for that indication. This combination—as is often the case, given synergistic interactive effects of different types of therapy and different classes of psychopharmacologic agents—was and has been effective for AB for years, and she has successfully incorporated the exercise part of her anti-panic (see Chap. 4) regimen into her daily activities.

Antidepressant Agents

A large number of psychotropic agents constitutes the second major "anti" subclass of psychopharmacotherapeutic medications, viz., "antidepressant agents." Also known historically as "mood elevators" and "thymoleptics," the biochemically based classifications of medications in this subclass have varied over the years, as have the approved indications for "antidepressant" agents. This point is especially true concerning the overlap of anxious and depressive symptomatology in presumably "depressed" individuals' (for whom antidepressant medications work well for such patients'/clients' symptoms) anxiety, and concerning both the general ineffectiveness for depressive symptoms in bipolar disorder and the induction of mania (the "switch process") in depressed patients/clients antidepressant medications may produce.

However, for present purposes, I will use predominant current nomenclature for the several types of antidepressant medications potentially prescribed by readers of this *Primer*. These include (1) Cyclic compounds (tricyclic, tetracyclic, heterocyclic, and polycyclic, referring to the biochemical molecular ring structures of these medications); (2) Mono-amino oxidase inhibitors (further divided into MAOa inhibitors, and MAOb inhibitors, depending on their pharmacologic properties; (3) Reuptake inhibitors of various types (Table 3.3); (4) Other miscellaneous preparations; and (5) Combination preparations. Without reiterating details and nuances of the *DSM-5* classifications and subclassifications, the main clinical indication for these antidepressant medications is major depressive disorder ("unipolar depression"), persistent depressive disorder (dysthymia), and other variants, but **not** bipolar depression (see below).

Table 3.3 delineates the several types of reuptake inhibitors among antidepressant agents, and Table 3.4 summarizes the overall subclasses of "antidepressant" psychopharmacotherapeutic medications.

Table 3.3 Types of neurotransmitter reuptake inhibitors (mostly antidepressant agents)

Neurotransmitter reuptake inhibitor class	Specific medications Generic name (Brand name)
Serotonin reuptake inhibitors (SRIs)	Citalopram (Celexa®) Escitalopram (Lexapro®) Paroxetine (Paxil®; PaxilER® [extended release]): at low dose Venlafaxine (Effexor®): at low dose Fluvoxamine (Luvox®): indicated for OCD Trazodone (Desyrel®) Vortioxetine (Trintellix®) Vilazodone (Viibryd®) Nefazodone (Serzone®): discontinued in 2003; equivalents may be available
Norepinephrine reuptake inhibitors (NRIs)	Desipramine (Norpramin®) Nortriptyline (Pamelor®) Atomoxetine (Strattera®): the only indicated non-stimulant for ADHD
SRIs/NRIs (mixed action)	Duloxetine (Cymbalta®, Irenka®) Venlafaxine (Effexor®): at usual dose Fluoxetine (Prozac®) Levomilnacipran (Fetzima®) Paroxetine (Paxil®; Paroxetine ER® [extended release]): at usual dose Clomipramine (Anafranil®): indicated for OCD Amitriptyline (Elavil®) Doxepin (Sinequan®; Adapin®) Imipramine (Tofranil®)
SRIs/DRIs (dopamine receptor inhibitors)	Sertraline (Zoloft®)

Adapted from Ghaemi (2019)

Generally, antidepressant psychopharmacotherapy is effective in about two-thirds of patients/clients, and more often in combination with other types of treatment (e.g., counseling/psychotherapy; see Chaps. 7 and 8). One longstanding technique to enhance that yield is "augmentation," or supplementation, of underlying psychopharmacotherapy—especially of tricyclic antidepressant medications—with a variety of agents. These agents include lithium compounds (at relatively low dosages), which are often effective, and electroconvulsive therapy (ECT; see Chap. 9) for individuals with treatment-resistant depression (TRD), non-responsive to psychopharmacotherapy.

Other augmentation strategies include triiodothyronine (T3, and other thyroid preparations, for thyroid replacement therapy, used off-label for antidepressant augmentation), tryptophan (an essential amino acid used off-label for antidepressant augmentation; see Chap. 6), methylphenidate (Ritalin® and others; see Chap. 4, section "Anti-ADHD Agents"), and pindolol (Visken® and others; a non-selective beta-blocker antihypertensive medication used off-label for antidepressant augmentation), all with lackluster to moderate treatment responses.

Table 3.4 Antidepressant agents

Cyclic compounds
  A. Tricyclics (TCAs)
    Amitriptyline (Elavil®, Etrafon®, and others)
    Clomipramine (Anafranil®)
    Desipramine (Norpramin® and others)
    Doxepin (Sinequan® and others)
    Imipramine (Tofranil® and others)
    Nortriptyline (Pamelor®, Aventyl®, and others)
    Protriptyline (Vivactil® and others)
    Trimipramine (Surmontil® and others)
  B. Other cyclic compounds (tetracyclic, bicyclic, heterocyclic, polycyclic)
    Amoxapine (Asendin®)
    Maprotiline (Ludiomil®)
    Mirtazapine (Remeron®)
    Venlafaxine (Effexor®)
    Desvenlafaxine (Pristiq®)

Monoamine oxidase inhibitors (MAOIs)
  A. MAO-As
    Isocarboxazid (Marplan®)
    Phenylzine (Nardil®)
    Tranylcypromine (Parnate®)
  B. MAO-Bs (see also section "Antiparkinsonian Agents," in Chap. 4, this book)
    Selegiline (Zelapar®; Emsam® patch [transdermal application]; Eldepryl®)

Selective serotonin reuptake inhibitors (SSRIs) and other reuptake inhibitors (Table 3.3)
  Citalopram (Celexa®)
  Escitalopram (Lexapro®)
  Fluoxetine (Prozac®)
  Paroxetine (Paxil®; Paxil ER®; and others)
  Sertraline (Zoloft®)
  Vilazodone (Viibryd®)
  Vortioxetine (Trintellix®)

Serotonin/norepinephrine agonist (SNA)
  Mirtazepine (Remeron®)

Serotonin antagonist/agonist (mixed)
  Buspirone (Buspar®)

Other agents
  Bupropion (Wellbutrin®): "stimulating" and similar in chemical structure to amphetamines, with mild dopamine and norepinephrine
  Nefazodone (Serzone®)
  Trazodone (Desyrel®)
  Ketamine (Spravato®; nasal spray; racemic ketamine infusion)

Combination preparations
  Amitriptyline (Elavil®) and perphenazine (Trilafon®): an antipsychotic; Triavil® and Etrafon® (no longer manufactured under these names: generic equivalents may be available)
  Amitriptyline (Elavil®) and Chlordiazepoxide (Librium®): an antianxiety agent; Limbitrol® (for mixed anxiety and depression)

With the wide variety of types and classes of psychopharmacologic entities comprising the "Antidepressant Agents," and the overlapping symptomatology among the various imprecise diagnostic categories to be treated by these agents, their use may be associated with a wide variety of undesirable ("side") effects. These effects, in turn, may be difficult to separate from symptomatology attributable to the condition being presumably treated, from symptomatology attributable to other co-occurring (comorbid) conditions or from a combination of all of these potential sources of undesirable effects. As with the earlier "Antianxiety Agents" section of this present chapter, I will not reiterate details of types and subtypes of the *DSM-5* classification of depressive disorders: The reader is referred to applicable parts of the *DSM-5* for that information.

Two case vignettes both illustrate psychopharmacotherapeutic approaches to individuals with major depressive disorder and with a variant of depression, respectively, and also illustrate a frequent mistake made in the treatment/management of such individuals.

AJ, a 62-year-old widow, presented to her psychiatric PA with chief complaints of a three-month history of initial and terminal insomnia, anorexia, and a seven-pound weight loss, pervasive "blues" improving somewhat as the day progressed, and a pervasive sense of worthlessness and hopelessness. The onset of these symptoms coincided with the death of her husband, with some feelings of blame and guilt that "the marriage could have been better." AJ had experienced a similar episode 23 years before, with the death of her mother; that short-lived episode remitted spontaneously, with counseling/psychotherapy treatment. AJ's older sister had been psychiatrically hospitalized in her 30s for a serious depressive illness, and responded well to a series of 10 electroconvulsive therapy (ECT) treatments. AJ's psychiatric PA prescribed supportive psychotherapy with a young empathetic female social worker and a clinical trial of trazodone (Desyrel®), both to address AJ's depression and her insomnia. After about three to four weeks of this combined treatment, AJ felt better and more optimistic, had more energy, slept better, and heaped praise on her psychotherapist and her psychopharmaco-therapist for "helping me so much, the combination of both of you. I've even gone back to yoga." AJ's improvement continued over the next nine months, to the present.

XY, a 37-year-old single stockbroker, remarked to his dentist that he had been experiencing "the blues" over about the past four months. This was possible concomitant with a downturn in his work, but "probably not. I've been through that before." His dentist referred him to a practicing prescribing clinical psychologist,[3] a "friend of a friend." That psychologist took a history, and prescribed fluoxetine (Prozac®), in that XY did not describe problems with insomnia. At first, XY told his psychologist that he felt "a little better." After about two weeks, however, XY did not keep an appointment, telephoned the psychologist two days later that "on a whim I picked up a woman in a bar, bought a Ferrari, drove to Minnesota, had the greatest sex ever, and I never want to come back." He eventually did return and

---

[3]This appointment took place in Baton Rouge, Louisiana, where licensed psychologists are permitted by law to prescribe psychotropic medications (i.e., "prescribing privileges") under certain circumstances and conditions. As of this writing, five states, Guam, the Indian Health Service (of the U.S. Public Health Service), and the U.S. military permit prescribing privileges for psychologists with specific training in psychopharmacology. The states are Idaho, Illinois, Iowa, Louisiana, and New Mexico, with efforts underway in additional states to grant psychologists' prescribing privileges.

revealed his history of several manicky episodes "a few years back," to his psychologist, who discontinued her patient's fluoxetine (Prozac®). The psychologist continued counseling/psychotherapy with XY, and eventually placed him on a clinical trial of lithium (see below), with the help of XY's primary care physician. XY returned to a baseline level of euthymia (normal range of mood and activity level) after a few weeks.

The first case ("AJ") is a straightforward example of a history and proper diagnosis of major depressive disorder, effectively treated with antidepressant psychopharmacotherapy and supportive counseling/psychotherapy. It also illustrates the trend in contemporary mental health care for counseling/psychotherapy with patients/clients as done by counselors and therapists of a variety of types (see Part II of this book) and for psychopharmacotherapy, as done by primary care NPs, PAs, physicians, and other prescribers.

The second case ("XY") illustrates the "switch process," in which antidepressant medication triggered a manic episode in an individual with a variant of depression called bipolar depression: In that situation, an individual's depressive episode (generally more common in individuals with bipolar disorder; see below, "Antimanic Agents") is part of the cycle pattern of mood fluctuation in bipolar disorder, and may respond to an antidepressant "push" by transitioning into a manic episode. This is what happened with XY, whose prior history of manic episodes and bipolar disorder had not been known to his treating psychologist until after his manic episode.

In concluding this section of this chapter, I emphasize the protean and variable types of chemical compounds that constitute "antianxiety agents" and "antidepressant agents." In addition to this resulting in multiple, overlapping, and variable undesirable ("side") effects, it also results in multiple uses and indications for these medications, both off-label and FDA-approved. Table 3.5 illustrates some of the latter.

Table 3.5 Approved (FDA) indications for uses of SSRIs and other drug classes

Major depression
Citalopram (Celexa®), escitalopram (Lexapro®), fluoxetine (Prozac®), paroxetine (Paxil®), and sertraline (Zoloft®); TCAs; SNRIs; MAOIs; others
Obsessive-compulsive disorder
Fluoxetine, fluvoxamine (Luvox®), paroxetine, and sertraline
Social anxiety disorder (social phobia)
Fluoxetine, paroxetine, and sertraline
Panic disorder
Paroxetine and sertraline; benzodiazepines (alprazolam [Xanax®]; clonazepam [Klonopin®]; others)
Generalized anxiety disorder
Escitalopram and paroxetine; benzodiazepines (all)
Post-traumatic stress disorder
Paroxetine and sertraline; benzodiazepines (not all)
Premenstrual dysphoric disorder
Fluoxetine and sertraline
Bulimia nervosa
Fluoxetine

Adapted from Black and Andreasen (2014)

Antimanic Agents

As psychopharmacologic agents for treating manic episodes in individuals, the term "antimanic" is intended as a short and focused one emphasizing individuals with mood **instability**: mood swings ("affective instability" or "mood instability"), which include both manic and depressive episodes of varying duration.

Unlike the other "anti" subclasses of agents in this classification system, "Antimanic Agents" are few in number: Lithium compounds, carbamazepine (Tegretol®), valproate (Depakote®; Depakene®), and lamotrigine (Lamictal®) are all FDA-approved for treatment of bipolar disorder. All except lamotrigine are believed to have a mechanism of action at the neurocellular level as a "second messenger" with neuroprotective effects. Three of the four (not including lithium compounds) are also classified as "novel anticonvulsants" (or antiseizure drugs, or antiepileptic drugs [AEDs]), which as a group were developed, beginning in the 1990s. Several other novel anticonvulsants are used off-label for treatment of bipolar disorder, with reported results comparable to those seen in comparable FDA-approved medications for that indication (e.g., carbamazepine [Tegretol®] and oxcarbazepine [Trileptal®]).

Table 3.6 lists these "Antimanic Agents" and their legal status (FDA-approved or off-label).

Table 3.6 Approved and off-label antimanic agents

Legal status			Agent
FDA-approved	Off-label	Not useful for psychiatric disorders	Generic name (Brand name)
X			Carbamazepine (Tegretol®)
X			Lamotrigine (Lamictal®)
X			Lithium carbonate preparations (Eskaleth®; Lithobid®)
X			Valproate (Depakene®; Depakote®)
	X		Gabapentin (Neurontin®)
	X		Oxcarbazepine (Trileptal®)
	X	X	Topiramate (Topamax®)
	X	X	Tiagabine (Gabitril®)
	X	X	Zonisamide (Zonegran®)

Concerning lithium compounds—a staple in the psychopharmacotherapy of mood instability—the undesirable ("side") effects of these agents are generally divided into mild and common (fine tremors, drowsiness and fatigue, memory problems, and excessive urination); moderate and less common (diarrhea, thirst, hypothyroidism, and more severe symptomatology of the mild type); and severe and unusual (cardiac electrical disturbances, hypothyroidism, and inappropriate antidiuretic hormone syndrome [IADH] and resulting fluid and electrolyte disturbances, among other). Severe or unusual side effects are often associated with inadvertent or deliberate overdose of lithium preparations.

Lithium levels typically are monitored via periodic lithium-level serum-blood-level determinations, and additional studies including periodic electrocardiograms (ECGs), complete blood counts (CBCs), thyroid function testing (TFTs), liver function testing (LFTs), urine studies, and others may also be done on an ongoing basis while an individual is taking this medication. In that way, both a patient's compliance with medication and possible development of side effects and undesired complications associated with chronic and ongoing lithium pharmacotherapy can be detected, tracked, and treated.

Anticonvulsants, mentioned earlier, are used primarily for the treatment of individuals with different types of seizure disorders. However, beginning with carbamazepine (Tegretol®) and valproate (valproic acid; Depakote® and Depakene®) as early as the 1960s, the mood-stabilizing effects of these drugs on individuals with bipolar disorder were recognized, and clinical research and practice into the mechanisms of action and usefulness of anticonvulsants in this area began and has continued. As is the case with any class of medications, the side effects of these mood-stabilizing anticonvulsants are based on their pharmacologic properties and may include dizziness, drowsiness, ataxia, somnolence, nausea, and vomiting, psychomotor slowing and dullness, decreased concentration, nervousness, tremor, and depression, among others.

Finally, in the context of other psychotropic medications used for bipolar disorder, other types of psychotropic medications, such as "atypical antipsychotics" (included in the "Antipsychotic Agents" subclass of this *Primer*'s classification system; see below) are FDA-approved for particular phases (e.g., acute mania; bipolar depression; maintenance) of the bipolar disorder cycle;[4] as adjunctive therapy for "Antimanic Agents;" for monotherapy (single-medication) therapy; for a combination of the two; and/or for pediatric use. The reader is referred to comprehensive references (above) and current internet sources for details of doses, treatment indications, FDA dose schedule, phases of cycle, prescribing practices, legal status, and the like, for these psychotropic medications.

Referring back to and continuing the case of "XY" to illustrate the psychopharmacotherapy of bipolar disorder, his story continued:

---

[4] The reader is referred to the *DSM-5* for further details and information about the classification, course, natural history, and progression of bipolar disorder.

After about four months on lithium psychopharmacotherapy and supportive psychotherapy/counseling, XY experienced the insidious onset of periodic palpitations and skipped heartbeats, erratic episodes of mild chest pain, weakness, and intermittent shortness of breath.

XY consulted his primary care physician, who examined him and did a battery of tests (including an electrocardiogram or ECG). The ECG showed erratic irregular beats of no specific pattern, and the doctor's recommendation was for XY to taper and discontinue his lithium medication. XY's psychiatric PA agreed, prescribed lamotrigine (Lamictal®), and tapered XY's lithium. After a stressful transition period, XY's new medication "kicked in" (his physician assistant's words), his cardiac symptoms stopped, and he remained stable over the next several months, to the present.

Antipsychotic Agents

Antipsychotic agents are also known as neuroleptics (from the Latin, "neuro-lysis" meaning "nerve-breaking"); "major tranquilizers" (an inaccurate term, based historically in contrast with "minor tranquilizers," or anxiolytics, as described above. The term "major tranquilizer" suggests that the principal effect of these medications is to sedate or "tranquilize" the patient/client taking them, in contrast to reducing or eliminating psychotic symptomatology); or—more recently, using a designation based on the presumed predominant biological mechanism of action of these agents—"dopamine blockers."

Antipsychotic agents are for the treatment of symptoms of thought disorders, or psychosis, the hallmark of which is symptomatology out of contact with reality. Such symptoms include so-called "positive symptoms" (e.g., delusions, defined as fixed and false beliefs which cannot be altered by logic or persuasion; hallucinations, defined as false de novo perceptions and sensations—in contrast to "illusions," which are perceptual distortions based on misinterpretations of actual stimuli, i.e., based on **something**, agitation, paranoia, occupational deterioration, and the like); and "negative symptoms" (apathy, withdrawal, depression, pessimism, and the like). These "negative" symptoms are said to be more effectively treated with the relatively recent type of antipsychotic medications called "atypical antipsychotics," or "second-generation" antipsychotics (SGAs) than with the older, traditional, conventional or "first-generation" antipsychotics (FGAs). These psychotic-level symptoms can also be associated with a wide range of underlying conditions, psychiatric and other.

Concerning the notion of "out of contact with reality," the concept of "neurotic" and "psychotic" levels of functioning is useful. "Neurotic"—a term derived from psychoanalytic theory, now considered outmoded by many, and not used in the *DSM-5*—refers to a level of functioning in which the patient/client is troubled, for example, tired, worried, anxious, tense, sad, and so forth, but functioning adequately: "Neurotics build castles in the air" (i.e., neurotic-level functioning). "Psychotic," on the other hand, refers to a level of functioning because of psychotic symptomatology which is not adequate: "Psychotics live in them" (i.e., psychotic-level functioning).

Psychotic-level disorders are classified in the *DSM-5* as "Schizophrenic Spectrum and Other Psychotic Disorders" (the chapter in the *DSM-5* which presents and discusses these disorders). The main disorders in this chapter are "Schizophrenia," "Schizoaffective Disorder," "Schizophreniform Disorder," "Delusional Disorder," and "Brief Psychotic Disorder," with several others listed, and with diagnostic criteria, details, associated features, and nuances given in the chapter. The reader is referred to that chapter in the *DSM-5* for that information and those details.

Concerning the psychopharmacotherapy of individuals with psychotic-level psychiatric disorders, and given that the desired antipsychotic effect for all of these agents is the same, the choice of a particular medication for a particular individual is based on optimizing the desired effect and minimizing the undesired effect of that medication. Since antipsychotic medications consist of a wide range of agents, which may produce adverse effects involving many organ systems, a practical approach to choosing and monitoring antipsychotic psychopharmacotherapy is given in a series of bulleted points in Table 3.7 followed by a list of potentially vulnerable organ systems, in Table 3.8. These tables, in turn, are followed by a list of antipsychotic medications currently in use, in Table 3.9. As with all of the "Anti" agents presented and discussed in this *Primer*, the reader is referred to applicable comprehensive textbooks and manuals, internet sources, and the like for details of dosing, dosing schedules, side effects, and other such information.

Table 3.7 Rational use of antipsychotic agents

1. *A high-potency conventional antipsychotic or one of the SGAs should be given as first-line treatment.*   SGAs are effective and well tolerated and have less potential to induce EPS.
2. *Second-line drug choices include the other conventional antipsychotics.*
3. *A drug trial should last 4-6 weeks.*   The trial should be extended when there is a partial response that has not plateaued and shortened when no response occurs or side effects are intolerable or unmanageable.   Aripiprazole, ziprasidone, or lurasidone may be the better choice in patients at risk for weight gain.   Quetiapine or aripiprazole may be favored when low EPS and low prolactin levels are desired.
4. *All antipsychotics should be started at a low dosage and gradually increased to fall within a therapeutic range.*   Evidence suggests that blood levels can help guide dosage adjustments for haloperidol and clozapine.
5. *There is little reason to prescribe more than one antipsychotic agent. Using two or more such drugs increases adverse effects and adds little clinical benefit.*
6. *Because of its risk of agranulocytosis and need for monitoring of the white blood cell count, clozapine should be reserved for patients with treatment-refractory illness.*
7. *Many patients can benefit from chronic antipsychotic administration.*   Patients should be carefully monitored for evidence of weight gain, glucose dyscontrol, and lipid abnormalities (metabolic syndrome).

Adapted from Hales et al. (2014)

Table 3.8 Organ systems potentially adversely affected by antipsychotic agents

Neurological
Metabolic
Hematologic
Genitourinary
Gastrointestinal
Cardiovascular
Endocrinologic

Adapted from Black and Andreasen (2014)

Table 3.9 Conventional (first-generation) and atypical (second-generation) antipsychotic agents

Category	Drug name (Brand name)
Conventional First-generation agents (FGAs)	
Phenothiazines Aliphatic Piperidines Piperazines	Chlorpromazine (Thorazine®) Thioridazine (Mellar®) Mesoridazine (Serentil®) Fluphenazine (Prolixin®) Fluphenazine decanoate Perphenazine (Trilafon®) Trifluoperazine (Stelazine®)
Thioxanthene	Thiothixene (Navane®)
Butyrophenone	Haloperidol (Haldol®)
Dihydroindolone	Molindone (Moban®; withdrawn in 2010)
Atypical Second-generation agents (SGAs)	Aripiprazole (Abilify®) Asenapine (Saphris®) Brexpiprazole (Rexulti®) Cariprazine (Vraylar®) Clozapine (Clozaril®) Lumateperone (Caplyta®) Lurasidone (Latuda®) Iloperidone (Fanapt®) Olanzapine (Zyprexa®) Quetiapine (Seroquel®) Paliperidone (Invega®) Risperidone (Risperdal®) Ziprasidone (Geodon®)

By way of illustration, the following case vignette includes such concerns in the treatment of psychotic-level patients as choice of medication, monitoring clinical progress, compliance/adherence, psychosocial issues, and others:

PR is a 57-year-old married, white female who works part-time as a librarian's assistant in her hometown of Everywhere and whose husband has worked in vehicle maintenance for the local Department of Public Works for the past 22 years. The couple has three children, ages 17, 23, and 25, of whom the youngest—a daughter—is still living at home. The family has lived in the same three-bedroom rented apartment for ten years. PR has a 23-year history of schizophrenic disorder (diagnosed then as "schizoaffective schizophrenia"), questionably associated with the birth of her second child and has been hospitalized in psychiatric facilities five times during those years.

Psychiatric treatment over the years has consisted of supportive psychotherapy—usually with a private psychiatrist—on an infrequent basis, neuroleptic medications, and support from her family.

The patient was hospitalized most recently the previous November for four weeks in a private facility following a period of rapid decompensation associated to some extent with losses in her life (specifically, her daughter's plans to leave home to attend college and her referral to a new psychiatrist after her previous psychiatrist of 10 years moved to California). Her hospitalization was uneventful and she was discharged in stable condition; the only possible problem during her hospitalization was the presence of mild rigidity, cog-wheeling in her arms and a slightly stiff gait; she was discharged on 2 mg. of benztropine mesylate (Cogentin®) by mouth, twice a day, which did not seem to be initially effective in management of these signs of extrapyramidal syndrome (EPS).

On February 11, 2011, PR was taken to the emergency room at Everywhere General Hospital at 11:00 p.m. by the Everytown Rescue Squad in a highly delusional and agitated state, with the additional findings of delirium: Disorientation (in all four parameters), complete memory loss, and a perception of "wiggly things crawling all over my body" (formication). Additional history was obtained from her husband regarding her pharmacotherapeutic management: Her new psychiatrist, Dr. Best, had been "juggling medications" for the past several months in an effort to arrive at the best combination for her and the patient herself had probably been inadvertently overdosing herself for the past several weeks. The patient had been increasingly forgetful and withdrawn over the past three weeks; the patient's current medication consists of 4 mg. of Risperdal®, by mouth, three times a day, and 6 mg. of benztropine mesylate (Cogentin®), by mouth, twice a day— increased over the months in an effort to control what Dr. Best felt was PR's increasing EPS. Dr. Best has been on vacation for one week.

This case vignette illustrates some of the complex interrelationships between psychotherapy, pharmacotherapy, family support, compliance/adherence to treatment plans, patient/client factors (here, specifically, the extent to which PR inadvertently or purposefully took too much medication ["overdosed"]), and other such factors, in keeping with the Epidemiologic Triangle model discussed earlier in this book. The case also illustrates the need to "think outside the box" in terms of complicating and overlapping neurologic conditions, such as dystonia, EPS, delirium, and withdrawal (apathy).

Finally, for present purposes, Table 3.10 summarizes advisable treatment practices to enhance treatment adherence/compliance to the extent possible. In the table, "long-acting injectables" (LAIs) refers to parenteral preparations of certain antipsychotic agents for depot injections which leech out over time into the patient's/client's body from the intramuscular depot injection site. The duration of action of different preparations is from weeks to months, as presented in Table 3.11.

Table 3.10 Treatment strategies to enhance patient/client adherence/compliance

Arrange for a convenient and uncomplicated dosing schedule
Provide patient/client education: discussion, patient package insert (PPI), etc.
Arrange for a convenient and uncomplicated dosing schedule
Minimize adverse effects, to the extent possible, taking into account medication factors (pharmacodynamic; pharmacokinetic), patient/client factors, and environmental factors (supportive home, denial of illness, etc.)
Follow-up and check for patient/client compliance/adherence (phone; pill counts)
Consider using long-acting injectable (LAI) preparations with appropriate patients/clients, where indicated

Table 3.11 First- and second-generation long-acting injectable (LAI) antipsychotics

	Medication	FDA-approved indications	Maintenance dose frequency (duration of action)
Conventional (First-generation) Antipsychotics	Bromperidol decanoate* Fluphenazine decanoate (Prolixin®) Flupenthixol decanoate (Fluanxol®) Haloperidol decanoate (Haldol decanoate*) Zuclopenthixol decanoate (Clopixol®; generic equivalent available in the U.S.)	Psychosis Psychosis Psychosis Psychosis Psychosis	Variable 2–3 weeks 1–4 weeks 3–4 weeks Several days for induction for antipsychotic action
Atypical (Second-generation) Antipsychotics	Aripiprazole LAI** (Abilify Maintena®) Aripiprazole lauroxil Olanzepine pamoate LAI (Zyprexa®) Paliperidone palmitate LAI (Invega Trinza®) Paliperidone palmitate (Invega Sustenna®) Paliperidone palmitate (3 mo. injections) (Invega Sustenna®) Risperidone LAI (Risperdal Consta®) Risperidone LAI for SQ (Perseris®)	Schizophrenia: Bipolar disorder Schizophrenia Schizophrenia Schizophrenia Schizophrenia Schizoaffective disorder Schizophrenia Schizophrenia: Bipolar disorder Schizophrenia	4 weeks 4 weeks 2–4 weeks 2–4 weeks 4 weeks 12 weeks 4 weeks 4 weeks

Adapted from Parmentier B. *Curr Psychiatry*. (2020)
[a]Used in Belgium, Italy, Germany, and the Netherlands
[b]LAI: "Long-acting injectable" medication formulation

A Note on References

Rather than burdening the reader with excessive and detailed references and citations in this *Primer*, given below are particularly useful selected references. In addition, other specific references and citations will be given in parentheses throughout the *Primer*. For further information and details about any topics presented and discussed in this book, the interested reader is referred not only to the following list of selected references, but also to applicable textbooks, monographs, electronic databases, print articles and materials, internet sources, and other applicable resources.

Selected References

- Black DW, Andreasen NC. Introductory textbook of psychiatry. 6th ed. American Psychiatric Publishing, Inc.; 2014. (A solid basic textbook of psychiatry.)
- Multiple Authors. Diagnostic and statistical manual of mental health disorders (*DSM-5*). 5th ed. American Psychiatry Association, Inc.; 2013. (This book is the controversial "bible" for primarily American and Canadian psychiatric diagnoses.)
- The comparable international work to the *DSM-5* is currently the 2019 International classification of diseases (*ICD-10*). 10th ed. World Health Organization. (The *ICD-11* was due for adoption in 2020.)
- Frances A. Saving normal: an insider's revolt against out-of-control psychiatric diagnosis, big pharma, and the medicalization of ordinary life. Harper Collins Publishers; 2013. (The subtitle says it all! See Chap. 4 in this *Primer*.)
- Ghaemi SN. Clinical psychopharmacology: principles and practice. Oxford University Press; 2019. (A scholarly, detailed, and lengthy overview of psychopharmacology, also covering social practice and research/methodologic aspects of the field.)
- Hales RE, Yudofsky ST, Roberts LW, editors, et al. The American Psychiatric Publishing textbook of psychiatry. 6th ed. American Psychiatric Publishing, Inc.; 2014. (A standard, detailed encyclopedic textbook tome, for reference. A seventh edition is available, copyright 2019, with updated coverage in a number of areas.)
- Harrington A. Mind fixers: psychiatry's troubled search for the biology of mental illness. W.W. Norton and Company; 2019. (A historical and scholarly review of the topic, including some of the same topics as *Saving Normal* listed above.)
- Puzantian T, Carlat DJ. Medication fact book for psychiatric practice. 6th ed. Carlat Publishing, LLC; 2020. (A very useful "cookbook" for psychotropic prescribing, conveniently organized and presented for the practitioner.)
- Watters E. Crazy like us: the globalization of the American psyche. Free Press; 2010. (Psychiatric diagnostic issues similar to those in *Saving Normal*, with an international focus.)

- Weil A. Mind over meds: know when drugs are necessary, when alternatives are better—and when to let your body heal on its own. Little, Brown and Company; 2017. (A balanced and holistic approach to pharmacology and psychopharmacology by the popular "guru" of these fields.)

Selected Internet References

With the surfeit of internet resources, websites of all imaginable types and quality, and numerous related electronic sources of information and data, the reader, clinician, researcher, and member of the public—patient/client or not—may easily become confused about where to go and what to accept in learning psychopharmacology and psychopharmacotherapy. In this vein, a productive way to navigate the bewildering array of such sources consists of dividing them into several categories, viz.

1. Refereed ("peer-reviewed;" "juried") scientific, technical, and professional journals, newsletters, and the like, including e-journals, e-newsletters, and other open-source e-publications. Selected examples include:

   - *Journal of Clinical Psychopharmacology* (peer-reviewed independent professional journal)
   - *Experimental & Clinical Psychopharmacology* (peer-reviewed professional journal of the American Psychological Association)
   - *Journal of Psychopharmacology* (peer-reviewed professional journal of the British Association for Psychopharmacology)
   - *Psychopharmacology* (Berlin/Heidelberg; Springer Publications)

2. Government and academic/research institutions, publications and e-publications, and associated websites. Selected examples include:

   - National Institute of Mental Health (NIMH) website, affiliated institutes, programs, centers, websites, and publications (electronic and print)
   - National Institute on Alcoholism and Alcohol Abuse (NIAAA) website, affiliated institutes, programs and centers, and websites and publications (electronic and print)
   - National Institute on Drug Abuse (NIDA) website, affiliated institutes, centers, programs and websites, and publications (electronic and print)
   - Canadian Centre on Substance Abuse (CCSA), affiliated programs and publications (electronic and print)
   - National Center on Addiction and Substance Abuse at Columbia University (NCASACU), programs and publications (electronic and print)

3. Journals, magazines, societies, and associated websites. Selected examples include:

   - *Psychology Today*

- *Scientific American*
- *Scientific American Mind*

As a practical matter, in researching particular topics electronically in psychopharmacology/psychopharmacotherapy, the logical rule—as with everything else—is to search for topic(s), keyword(s), and the like on a search engine, then to narrow the search with entries given by the search engine. An important factor to keep in mind here is the reliability, accuracy, and quality of the source: Sources from (1) and (2)—above—are considered more reliable than those in (3), generally. Those in (3), in turn, are generally considered more reliable than personal blogs, newsletters, product websites, company websites, and the like.

Chapter 4
The Sixteen "Minor Anti-s"

The term "minor" in the context of this *Primer* is not intended to be synonymous with "trivial" or "unimportant." For an individual afflicted with any of these conditions, the associated symptomatology and distress can be serious, or "major." Rather, the term "minor" as used in this system of "Major," "Minor," "Anti" psycho-pharmacotherapeutic is intended as a reflection of the prevalence of the conditions treated by their various "Anti" agents, and the frequency of prescribing professionals treating these conditions. In that sense, the unifying factor of the "Anti" classification scheme, or taxonomy does not pertain to common, or linked, pathophysiology of the conditions treated by the "Anti" agents, nor to common, or linked, mechanisms of action of the "Anti" agents themselves. Rather, as also discussed in Chap. 1, the unifying factor of the several "Anti" agents discussed in this *Primer* is the manifestational *symptomatology* from the underlying diagnosis, reduced or eliminated by the particular "Anti" agent.

The importance of an accurate *diagnosis* cannot be underestimated in this context, especially in view of the considerable overlap of symptomatology among different psychiatric conditions (The "differential diagnosis" of psychotic-level symptoms, for example, in schizophrenia and Parkinson's disease—discussed in upcoming sections of this *Primer*—illustrate this point.)

Anti-addiction Agents

The first of the "Anti-agents" to be discussed in this chapter are "Anti-addiction Agents" including reference to "medication-assisted treatment" or "MAT" (also discussed in Chap. 5).

As a treatment modality in health care, psychopharmacotherapeutic approaches to the treatment and management of addiction, substance abuse, and chemical dependency (which terms are used interchangeably here and are also discussed in

D. P. Greenfield, *Psychopharmacology for Nonpsychiatrists*, https://doi.org/10.1007/978-3-030-82507-2_4

Chap. 5) are relatively young, having begun with the use of disulfiram as an aversive agent to the pharmacologic treatment of alcoholism in the 1950s. This was followed by methadone in the 1960s and going forward, as a blocking agent to the euphorigenic effects of heroin and other opioids (i.e., *not* as an analgesic—"Anti-pain"— medication; see below in this chapter). Subsequent pharmacologic aversive, antagonistic, or blocking agents were developed over the ensuing years, for a variety of addictions and dependencies, such as nicotine addiction, addiction to heroin and other opioids, cocaine addiction, and alcoholism, in the 1980s, 1990s, and 2000s.

In addition to chemical dependencies ("Substance Use Disorders," in *DSM-5* parlance), the several fields of addiction treatment have come to recognize the so-called "Behavioral (i.e., not chemical) Addictions" as involving the same types of neurobiological mechanisms of action as chemical dependencies, and therefore a legitimate focus of attention for the fields of addiction treatment. Table 4.1 gives examples of the "Behavioral Addictions."

Table 4.1 Examples of behavioral addictions

Computer-based addictions
Internet gaming
Internet surfing
Internet pornography
Texting and emailing
Exercise
Food and eating disorders (see Chap. 4 of this book)
Kleptomania
Love
Sex
Shopping
Tanning
Work
Cutting

For present purposes—with the exception of some eating and feeding disorders—the principal overall treatment approach for the "Behavioral Addictions" is behavioral. This may include the various behavioral therapies (see Chaps. 7 and 8), family therapy, and psychopharmacotherapy with anti-depressant medications (e.g., some SSRIs for bulimic disorders, both FDA-approved and off-label), especially in situations where depression is present. Otherwise, since psychopharmacotherapy beyond symptomatic relief is not generally a significant part of the treatment of behavioral disorders, no further discussion of psychopharmacotherapy for behavioral disorders will follow.

However, the notion of symptomatic relief of "target symptoms" associated with the addictions and their often comorbid, or co-occurring, conditions, leads to the classification of "Anti-addiction Agents" into two parts. They are (1) psychopharmacotherapy to address, or counter, or block mechanisms of action of specific drugs of abuse and (2) psychopharmacotherapy of "target symptoms" attributable to drugs of abuse. The former approach is called medication-assisted treatment, or MAT, and the latter approach includes the types of psychopharmacotherapy covered in this *Primer*.

The rationale behind pharmacotherapy for the addictions involves the use of psychotropic agents as a substitute (i.e., a pharmacologic competitor *agonist*) for the addictive substance, with a more desirable main effect and side effect profile than that of the substance of abuse. Substituting methadone for street heroin is one example. Such drugs may also serve as a *partial* substitute (*a partial agonist*) for the addictive substance, such as nicotine replacement polacrilex gum. They might also serve as an antagonist, or blocking agent (to counter undesirable effects of the addictive substance, induce withdrawal or a withdrawal-like state, initiate detoxification, and produce an aversive experience for the user); examples are disulfiram (Antabuse®), naloxone (Narcan®), or naltrexone (Revia®) for opioid use. These drugs might also serve as anti-withdrawal agents (to reduce the discomfort and likelihood of convulsions, seizures, and delirium tremens); examples include benzodiazepines and anti-anxiety drugs and anti-convulsants to treat alcohol and other sedative-hypnotic withdrawal. Another use of these types of drugs is as anti-craving agents to reduce the drive and compulsion of an addict to seek the desired drug or medication. Finally, these drugs might serve as psychotropic medications or drugs to treat symptoms arising from comorbid, or co-occurring, psychiatric disorders in the substance-abusing patient with such psychiatric disorders.

Table 4.2 displays the above points in terms of the pharmacologic properties and mechanisms of action, along with examples of these medications. Table 4.3 presents specific anti-addiction agents in terms of their roles and indications in current concepts of medication-assisted treatment (MAT).

Table 4.2 Anti-addiction agents and properties

Drug of addiction	Pharmacologic property	Examples of medication
Alcohol	Agonists (substitute)	None
	Partial agonists	None
	Antagonists	Disulfiram (Antabuse®)
	Anti-withdrawal (detoxification) agents	Benzodiazepines; anti-convulsants
	Anti-craving agents	Naltrexone (Revia®; Vivitrol® LAI*)
	Concomitant treatment agents	Acamprosate (Campral®)
Cocaine	Agonists (substitute)	None
	Partial agonists	None
	Antagonists	None
	Anti-withdrawal (detoxification) agents	None (not a major clinical problem)
	Anti-craving agents	None
	Concomitant treatment agents	Varies
Nicotine	Agonists (substitute)	Nicotine substitution, polacrilex gum, patch, aerosol
	Partial agonists	None
	Antagonists	Mecamylamine
	Anti-withdrawal (detoxification) agents	Bupropion (Zyban®)
	Anti-craving agents	Nicotine substitution, bupropion
	Concomitant treatment agents	Varies
Opiates/ opioids	Agonists (substitute)	Methadone, LAAM
	Partial agonists	Buprenorphine and congeners
	Antagonists	Naltrexone (Revia®; Vivitrol® LAI*); Naloxone (Narcan®); Methadone
	Anti-withdrawal (detoxification) agents	Clonidine (Catapres®; Lofexidine); Buprenorphine

Adapted and updated from Kleber (1999), CME Symposium
*LAI: "Long-acting injectable" medication formulation

Table 4.3 Medication-assisted treatment (MAT)

For opioid addiction (opioid use disorder or OUD)
Methadone
Naltrexone (IR and L-A [Vivitrol,® injectable])
Buprenorphine (Subutex®; Suboxone® [buprenorphine + naloxone]; other short- and long-acting preparations)
For alcohol addiction (alcohol use disorder or AUD)
Disulfiram (Antabuse®)
Acamprosate (Campral®)
Naltrexone (Revia®)
For smoking (tobacco products)
Nicotine replacement therapy (patches, polacrilex gum, others) and vaping replacement therapy
Varenicycline (Chantix®)
Bupropion (Zyban® for smoking, specifically)

In therapeutic work with addicts and alcoholics, several practical points ought to be made:

- The heterogeneous agents and medications that comprise this class vary widely in their own pharmacologic actions and properties and may initially be associated with any side effect that can affect the central nervous system (CNS). The healthcare practitioner should know if the patient/client is taking or has taken any of these medications in order to assess whether symptoms attributed to other experiences may in fact be due to medication effects.
- A patient/client taking these medications for treatment of addiction may or may not be adherent/compliant with the treatment regimen. Depending on the extent of such adherence/compliance, nonspecific CNS symptomatology (such as discomfort, depression, agitation, excitement, irritability, and so forth) may be the result of complete or partial nonadherence/noncompliance and may erroneously be attributed to other experiences. It behooves the healthcare practitioner not only to inquire about whether the patient/client is taking prescribed anti-addiction medications but also about the extent to which the patient/client is taking the medication as prescribed.
- Finally, given the chronic and relapsing nature of the addictions and the nonspecific psychological/psychiatric symptomatology associated with relapses, such symptomatology in those situations may be erroneously attributed by the patient/client to life events and experiences, to prescribed medications, or to a combination of both, rather than to the true cause of such symptomatology—namely a relapse into active addiction and its accompanying symptoms.

A number of the points made in this "Anti-addiction Agents" section of this chapter will be revisited in Chap. 5, as mentioned above.

Anti-aggression Agents

As a practical matter, most aggression and violence associated with psychiatric disorders, however broadly interpreted, are not amenable to psychopharmacotherapeutic intervention. Aggression and violence are not psychiatric/neuropsychiatric "diseases" or "disorders" per se, but in certain cases, they may be signs/symptoms of underlying psychiatric disorders themselves. In those disorders in which aggressive and violent intentions, tendencies, or behaviors are, or may be, manifestations of the psychiatric conditions themselves, then psychopharmacotherapeutic intervention may be indicated. For that reason, proper diagnosis of a potential underlying psychiatric condition—as is always the case in clinical practice of any type—is paramount. Table 4.4 presents psychiatric disorders and conditions in which aggression and violence may be part of the clinical picture.

Table 4.4 Psychiatric, neuropsychiatric, and medical/ neurologic conditions and disorders with associated aggressive and violent symptomatology	
	Autism spectrum disorders (ASD)
	Neurocognitive disorders
	Conduct disorders
	Disruptive mood regulation disorders
	Intermittent explosive disorder (IED)
	Medical/neurologic conditions
	Oppositional defiant disorder (ODD)
	Personality disorders
	Schizophrenia and other psychotic disorders
	Adapted from Hales et al. (2014)

A variety of psychotropic medications from a variety of "Anti-agents" may be used for aggressive and violent symptoms as a manifestation of an underlying psychiatric disorder. These agents include anti-psychotic medications (aripiprazole [Abilify®] and risperidone [Risperdal®]) and anti-ADHD agents (methylphenidate [Ritalin®] and atomoxetine [Strattera®]). Under some circumstances, some SSRIs for anxiety and the driven repetitive behavior (e.g., rocking) seen in autism may also be useful. Behavioral interventions based on principles of operant conditioning are generally the most effective treatment modality and are the starting point for treatment and management of individuals with autism spectrum disorder (ASD).

The constellation in *DSM-5* of "disruptive impulse control and conduct disorders" includes a wide variety of conditions in which, as the designation implies, a number of "*DSM-5* Disorders" is represented. These include, in turn, neurodevelopmental disorders (ADHD), bipolar disorders, obsessive-compulsive disorder (OCD) and related conditions, substance use disorders (SUDs), and others. In situations in which aggressive/violent and related symptomatology arises as "target symptoms" from the underlying psychiatric disorder, or condition, applicable psychopharmacotherapy may be used, as clinically indicated for given cases.

Disruptive mood regulation disorder (DMRD), a new formal diagnostic designation in the *DSM-5*, like conduct disorder and others in this constellation, has aggression and out-of-control behaviors as a core sign/symptom. Specific psychopharmacotherapy for this condition has not been identified at this point, although in cases in which such symptoms as withdrawal, lethargy, and apathy predominate, then "activating" (non-sedating) anti-depressant agents may be indicated. Conversely, in cases in which agitation, aggression, irritability, and the like, predominate, then calming and sedating anti-depressant agents may be indicated.

Given the current state-of-the-art-and-science—in psychiatry and neuropsychiatry generally—that target symptom relief is the goal, then the goal for psychopharmacotherapy is first to identify "target symptoms" for this and any other psychiatric disorder condition (except, perhaps, some neurocognitive disorders) and to identify a psychopharmacologic agent with the ability to ameliorate the symptomatology.

Similarly, schizophrenia and other psychotic disorders may present out-of-control aggressive, violent, and actively psychotic "target" signs and symptoms often amenable to psychopharmacotherapy, with the "positive symptoms" (see Chap. 3) being considered generally amenable to conventional ("first-generation") and atypical ("second-generation") anti-psychotic medications, and "negative symptoms" (see Chap. 3) being considered generally amenable to atypical ("second-generation") anti-psychotic agents.

Finally, for present purposes, as a diagnostic category, or entity, "Personality Disorders" are perhaps the most "manifestational" in symptomatology and the least "causal" (see Chap. 2) in terms of causation, etiology, or pathogenesis of all psychiatric/neuropsychiatric conditions. The psychopharmacotherapeutic approach to these conditions, therefore, relies on identifying those personality disorders with the greatest overt "target" symptomatology potentially amenable to dulling, or amelioration. Examples include psychotic-level symptomatology in schizotypal disorder (amenable to "Antipsychotic Agents") and florid irritability, tension, and aggression in borderline personality disorder (amenable to "Anti-psychotic Agents" and to "Antianxiety Agents"). Even so, beneficial treatment effects of psychopharmacotherapy for individuals with borderline personality disorder are considered moderate, at best. Table 4.5 illustrates that point.

Table 4.5 Effectiveness of psychopharmacotherapy for personality disorders

Personality disorder	Effectiveness of psychopharmacotherapy
Cluster A (odd or eccentric)	
Paranoid	Uncertain
Schizoid	Not helpful
Schizotypal	Moderate (for treating associated "target symptoms")
Cluster B (dramatic, emotional or erratic)	
Antisocial	Not helpful
Borderline	Moderate (for treating associated "target symptoms")
Histrionic	Not helpful
Narcissistic	Not helpful
Cluster C (anxious or fearful)	
Avoidant	Uncertain
Dependent	Not helpful
Obsessive-compulsive	Not helpful

Adapted from Hales et al. (2014)

Anti-appetite Agents

Since the publication of an earlier version of this section of this chapter in 2009, the fields of clinical nutrition, primary care medicine, and mental health care have evolved considerably to include diet and exercise, weight control, appetite suppression, treatment of obesity and eating disorders, holistic medical care, complementary and alternative medicine (CAM; see Chap. 6 of the *Primer*), and other related topics.

A full discussion of these areas is well beyond the scope of this section of the chapter. In this section, however, I will focus on currently used medications for appetite management, in the context of a comprehensive and holistic approach to weight management. In the words of a prominent holistic dental practitioner, "If you diet, exercise, floss your teeth regularly, and don't smoke, you'll live forever!"

Appetite suppressants, "anorectics" or "Anti-appetite Agents" for present purposes, are the sixth of the 20 "Anti-s" in this classification system. As the name suggests, these medications are intended for use in weight loss and weight management. Within the "Anti" class are essentially two subtypes, (1) stimulants/psychostimulants (e.g., amphetamines and related compounds) and (2) metabolic agents (e.g., orlistat [Xenical®]). Table 4.6 presents these two subtypes and prescription and OCT medications currently available.

Table 4.6 Stimulant and non-stimulant appetite suppressants

Drug class	Medication	Mode of action
Stimulant/ psychostimulant	*Amphetamine* (Biphetamine®; Adderall®*)	CNS appetite suppression
	Fenfluramine (Pondimin®; removed from the market in 1998, in combination with Phentermine as Fen-Phen®)	CNS appetite suppression
	Mazindol (removed from the market in 2008)	CNS appetite suppression
	Methamphetamine (Desoxyn®)	CNS appetite suppression
	Phendimetrazine (various preparations)	CNS appetite suppression
	Phentermine (Adipex-P®)	CNS appetite suppression
	Sibutramine (Meridia®; removed from the market in 2010)	CNS appetite suppression
Other mechanisms	*Glucomannan* (OTC)	Inhibit digestion
	Guar gum (OTC)	Inhibit digestion
	Liraglutide (Saxenda®)	Mimic satiety
	Lorecaserin (Belviq®; removed from the market in 2020)	Mimic satiety
	Naltrexone/bupropion (Contrave®)	Anti-craving
	Phentermine/topiramate (Qsymia®)	CNS appetite suppression
	Rimonabant (Acomplia®; removed from the market in 2008)	Cannabinoid receptor antagonism

*Adderall®, or mixed amphetamine salts (MAS), is an amphetamine compound **not** indicated for appetite suppression. Its use is as an "Anti-ADHD Agents," discussed later in this chapter

The use of these medications for weight management and control has been controversial over the years, in large part due to the potentially addictive properties of psychostimulants and their legal status as Controlled Dangerous Substances (CDS) for most of them, with abuse and diversion potential. Nevertheless, to the extent that such psychopharmacotherapeutic agents are indicated and used for weight management, current professional acceptance in healthcare dictates that these medications be used on a short-term basis as part of a comprehensive, balanced clinical program of diet, exercise, good sleep, hygiene, good dental care, and other such healthy practices. The non-stimulant appetite suppressants—Qsymia® (phentermine and topiramate), Saxenda® (liraglutide), Contrave® (naltrexone/bupropion), and the OTC and other such preparations—are considered appropriate for long-term use.

Since a common feature of the stimulant/psychostimulant medications is their stimulating (speeding) quality, patients/clients should be educated about that predominant effect when these medications are prescribed and followed over time.

In the sections of this chapter on "Anti-ADHD Agents" and in Chap. 5 stimulants/psychostimulants will be discussed further.

Anti-attention Deficit Hyperactivity Disorder (ADHD) Agents

In his iconoclastic *Saving Normal: An Insider's Revolt Against Out-of-Control Psychiatric Diagnosis, DSM-5, Big Pharma, and the Medicalization of Ordinary Life* (2015), Allen Frances, M.D., former Professor and Chairperson of the Department of Psychiatry and Behavioral Medicine at Duke University School of Medicine, and Chairperson of the *DSM-IV* (the predecessor *Diagnostic and Statistical Manual of Mental Disorders* to the present *DSM-5*) Task Force, wrote about himself and his own possible ADHD diagnosis.

In the chapter entitled "Attention Deficit Disorder Runs Wild," of *Saving Normal*.[1] Dr. Frances described on one occasion having left his car at an airport while on a business trip, and not remembering its location when he returned. He had initially not paid attention to where he had left the car. The story ends happily, but Dr. Frances raises the question of whether his behavior warranted a formal diagnosis of ADHD: "My wife…unemphatically claims my lack of attention to the needs and errands of everyday life reflect willful avoidance rather than diagnosable mental disorder…"

But in this vein, Dr. Frances then questions the reportedly rapid recent increase in the prevalence of the formal ADHD diagnosis ("…an amazing 10 percent of kids now qualify…"). He offers a number of possible explanations for this prevalence, concluding that "…there is no reason to think the kids have changed, it is just the labels have…"

Without taking a position on this controversial condition, this present section of "Anti-ADHD Agents," in this chapter about the "Minor Anti-s," presents and discusses the basics of ADD (attention deficit disorder) and ADHD (attention deficit hyperactivity disorder) and the principal psychopharmacotherapeutic agents currently used in treatment of these conditions. As with "Anti-appetite Agents," most of these medications are stimulants/psychostimulants by drug class, potentially posing the same problems with abuse, dependence, and diversion (i.e., from prescribers' practices) as when they are used for other conditions or indications (see Chap. 5).

The *DSM-5*, for practical purposes, distinguishes between two main diagnostic features which give rise to the nomenclature and the term "attention deficit hyperactivity disorder," or ADHD. These features are *inattention* and *hyperactivity* (the *DSM-5* also discusses *impulsivity*, but that feature is not incorporated into the ADHD nomenclature). In terms of the life cycle, hyperactivity generally precedes inattention, starting in childhood, and in some cases, proceeding into the adult years. Population surveys indicate that the prevalence of ADHD in the general population is about 5% in children and about 2.5% in adults.

---

[1] For an even more iconoclastic and vehement treatment of these topics, see Watters E. *Crazy like us: the globalization of the American psyche*. Free Press; 2010.

For practical purposes, anti-ADHD agents may be classified into three subcategories, viz., (1) Methylphenidate and congeners; (2) Dexmethylphenidate (the dextro-isomer of methylphenidate); (3) Mixed amphetamine salts (MAS); and (4) Non-stimulant medications. The paradoxical effects of the stimulants/psychostimulants on children and adults with ADHD—the calming and organizing effects on the aggressive, irritable, distracted, and disorganized features, whether the inattentive, hyperactive, or combined types of ADHD—are counterintuitive, and are the basis for the positive results often seen in ADHD psychopharmacotherapy. Table 4.7 lists medications commonly used for ADHD psychopharmacotherapy, according to the three subcategories just noted.

Table 4.7 Anti-ADHD agents

1a. Methylphenidate formulations	2. Dextroamphetamine formulations
Generic (*IR*) (3–4 hours)	*DestroStat* (*IR*) (3–5 hours)
Methylin (*IR*) (3–4 hours)	*Dexedrine* (*IR*) (3–5 hours)
Methylin ER (6–8 hours)	*Generic* (*IR*) (3–5 hours)
Ritalin (*IR*) (3–4 hours)	*LiquADD* (3–5 hours) (dextroamphetamine sulfate)
Ritalin SR (6–8 hours)	*Dexedrine Spansule* (6–8 hours)
Generic SR (6–8 hours)	*Dextroamphetamine ER* (6–8 hours)
Metadate ER (6–8 hours)	*Vyvanse* (12–14 hours) (lisdexamfetamine dimesylate)
Ritalin LA (8–10 hours)	
Metadate CD (6–8 hours)	
Concerta (12 hours)	
Daytrana (transdermal)	
1b. Dexmethylphenidate formulations	
Focalin (3–4 hours)	
Ceneric (3–4 hours)	
Focalin XR (10–12 hours)	
3. Mixed amphetamine salts (MAS)	4. Non-stimulants
Adderall (*IR*) (3–5 hours)	*Atomexetine* (Strattera®; NRI)
Generic (*IR*) (3–5 hours)	*Bupropion* (Wellbutrin®; off-label for ADHD)
Adderall XR capsule (10–12 hours)	*Clonidine XR* (Kapvay®)
Generic (*XR*) (10–12 hours)	*Guanfacine ER* (Intuniv®; α-agonist [alpha-adrenoceptor agonist])
	Guanfacine IR (Tenex®; α-agonist [alpha-adrenoceptor agonist]; not approved for children)
	Modafinil (Provigil®; not approved for children)

Key: *ER* extended release, *IR* immediate release, *NRI* norepinephrine reuptake inhibitor

As a practical matter, the predominant current use of anti-convulsant agents (or antiepileptic drugs [AEDs], or anti-seizure drugs) in psychiatric practice is for bipolar disorder (see section "Antimanic Agents," Chap. 3), either alone or in combination with other psychotropic agents (such as atypical anti-psychotic agents) to address various phases of the disorder, although other conditions (such as anxiety disorders and substance use disorders) have been treated with good results by anti-convulsant agents, as well. Table 4.8 delineates these phases in bipolar disorder in which anti-convulsant psychopharmacotherapy has a role.

Although more likely used in neurology practice for treating patients with seizure disorders of a variety of types, lithium and two anti-convulsants (valproic acid [Depakote®] and carbamazepine [Tegretol®]) have been used in the treatment of bipolar disorder (or manic-depressive disorder, as the condition was known then) since as long ago as the 1960s, and beginning in the 1990s, several novel anti-convulsants have been developed and used in various aspects of psychiatric practice. Table 4.9 gives a summary of these agents and their other (i.e., other than for treating seizures) clinical indications in psychiatric practice.

Table 4.8 Phases of bipolar disorder treated with anti-convulsants and other agents

Phase of illness	Psychopharmacotherapeutic approach
Manic episodes	Anti-psychotic agents, enhanced with mood stabilizers (e.g., risperidone [Risperdal®] with lithium, and lorazepam [Ativan®] as needed)
Bipolar depression	Symbyax® (fluoxetine [Prozac®] and olanzapine [Zyprexa®]), quetiapine [Seroquel®], lurasidone [Latuda®], and cariprazine [Vraylar®], (FDA-approved); lithium compounds, lamotrigine [Lamictal®], and aripiprazole [Abilify®], with augmentation with bupropion [Wellbutrin®], probably least likely to cause a manic switch (off-label use)
Bipolar treatment maintenance	Lithium, lamotrigine [Lamictal®], valproic acid [Depakote®], carbamazepine [Tegretol®]

Table 4.9 Anti-convulsant agents

Indications	Agents
Anti-convulsants used in psychiatry: older agents	Carbamazepine (Tegretol®; others[a]) Oxcarbazepine (Trileptal®; others) Valproic acid (Depakote®; Depakene®; others)
Anti-convulsants used in psychiatry: novel anti-convulsants	Gabapentin (Neurontin®; others) Pregabalin (Lyrica®, CDS-V; off-label for neuropathic pain and anxiety) Tiagabine (Gabitril®; off-label for anxiety and pain) Topiramate (Topamax®; others)
Novel anti-convulsants not used in psychiatry	Levetiracetam (Keppra®; others) Vigabatrin (Sabril®; others) Zonisamide (Zonegran®; others)

[a]As also described earlier in this book, several brands with different brand or trade names by different manufacturers are available for many medications of all types, once the compound's patent life has expired. "Others" in this Table indicates that alternative brand names are available for the basic compound, also known as the "generic equivalent." At the time of this writing, pregabalin (Lyrica®) was under patent protection

As noted above, other psychiatric conditions in which the novel anti-convulsants may have a role in treatment include anxiety disorders (see Chap. 3) and substance use disorders (see Chap. 5). Examples of these medications and their indicated conditions are pregabalin (Lyrica®), which seems useful as a cross-reactive agent in tapering and discontinuing benzodiazepines, and in reducing neuropathic (e.g., peripheral diabetic neuropathy) pain; topiramate (Topamax®) as an adjunct for alcohol dependence and weight loss (in virtually any condition); and gabapentin (Neurontin®) for alcohol dependence and anxiety.

Concerning side effects of the novel anti-convulsants, while they are in general less toxic than older anti-convulsants, these medications as a class carry a "black box" (FDA drug class) warning for increased risk of suicidal thoughts and behaviors and have to be monitored carefully in patients for that reason. In addition, prescriptions for both pregabalin (Lyrica®) and gabapentin (Neurontin®) are frequently diverted from clinical practices and abused, prompting some states to mandate reporting of them (like "Controlled Dangerous Substances," or CDS; see Chap. 5) to some states instituting Prescription Drug Monitoring Programs (PDMPs)—as in New Jersey—to control their misuse and spread.

Anti-dementia Agents

Known also as "cognition enhancers," these agents are intended to slow the progression of dementing diseases, such as Alzheimer's disease, especially in the elderly population. Generally, such slowing will last 6–12 months, after which the decline in memory and progression of other secondary signs and symptoms (such as agitation, restlessness, wandering ["sundowning"], irritability, hostility, dysphonia, mood swings, and depression) will resume. At that point, the efficacy of using another anti-dementia to re-establish a plateau in memory loss in unclear. If the course of treatment is interrupted, cognitive decline will be accelerated and not likely to regain the previous level of cognitive functioning if resumed.

Recognizing the prevalence and difficulty of both the primary memory decline and the secondary signs and symptoms of dementing diseases, Table 4.10 presents the principal classes of medications useful in ameliorating these signs and symptoms, along with their mechanisms of action and clinical indications. Some of these classes and medications have already been discussed, and others will be discussed later in this *Primer*.

Table 4.11 presents a list of miscellaneous agents of a variety of types potentially useful in a myriad of ways for treating patients with dementias.

Table 4.10 Anti-dementia agents useful for primary and secondary signs and symptoms of dementia

Class of medication	Examples	Clinical indications
1. Primary signs and symptoms (memory loss)		
Cholinesterase inhibitors (and some with other cholinergic actions)	Donepezil (Aricept®)	Mild, moderate, severe Alzheimer's dementia (dose-dependent)
	Galantamine (Razadyne®)	Mild to moderate Alzheimer's dementia
	Rivastigmine (Exelon®)	Mild to moderate Alzheimer's and Parkinsonian dementia
	Rivastigmine (Exelon Patch®)	Mild to moderate Alzheimer's and Parkinsonian dementia
N-Methyl-D-aspartate (NMDA) receptor antagonists	Memantine (Namenda®)	Moderate to severe Alzheimer's dementia
	Memantine ER (Namenda XR®)	Moderate to severe Alzheimer's dementia
	Memantine ER/donepezil (Namzaric®)	Moderate to severe Alzheimer's dementia (for individuals on both medications, a combination single-dose agent)
(2) Secondary signs and symptoms		
Selective serotonin reuptake inhibitors (SSRIs)	Escitalopram (Lexapro®) Sertraline (Zoloft®)	Agitation, hostility, irritability, restlessness Agitation, hostility, irritability, restlessnessS
Serotonin-norephedrine agonists	Mirtazapine (Remeron®)	Insomnia, depression
Benzodiazepines (see "Antianxiety Agents")	Lorazepam (Ativan®) and other short-acting agents	Use on a short-term basis; associated with excess sedation, memory loss; low doses
Anti-psychotics (see "Anti-psychotic Agents")	Risperidone (Risperdal®): *not* in Parkinson's patients	Low-dose; *be aware* of the FDA "black box" warning (2005) against use of anti-psychotics in the elderly because of increased risk of stroke (CVA)
	Quetiapine (Seroquel®), clozapine (Clozaril®), or pimavanserin (Nuplazid®) for Parkinson's patients	*Only* for treating psychotic symptoms; *monitor* carefully
Serotonin-norephedrine agonists	Gabapentin (Neurontin®) Lamotrigine (Lamictal®) Oxcarbazepine (Trileptal®) Valproic acid (Depakote®) Lithium preparation	Manicky symptomatology; stabilization and calming; monitor carefully for lithium and other toxicity

Adapted from Puzantian and Carlat (2020)

Table 4.11 Other agents of use in dementia

Acetaminophen (Tylenol®) for pain, often underdiagnosed in dementia patients. Opioids (low dose) can also be useful, recognizing confusion and potential for falls; monitor carefully.
Trazodone (Desyrel®), for agitation and insomnia, at low doses.
Prazosin (Minipress®, others). Originally an antihypertensive medication, used in dementia patients for agitation, nightmares, and related PTSD symptomatology (see section "Anti-trauma Agents"). Monitor blood pressure and sensorial carefully.
Clonidine patch (Catapres®, others). Another antihypertensive agent, originally used in dementia patients for agitation and anxiety, and useful ensuing adherence/compliance (transdermal delivery system). Monitor blood pressure and sensorium carefully.
Dronabinol (Marinol®), a cannabinoid preparation for diminishing weight loss in AIDS and nausea from chemotherapy, off-label use in agitation with dementia patients.

Adapted from Puzantian and Carlat (2020)

Last—but probably most important for these frail demented individuals, considering the potential adverse ("side") effects of the wide range of "anti-dementia" medications—the treating professional should practice nonpharmacologic interventions first, such as individual and group counseling/psychotherapy (especially for depressed individuals with dementia), art and music therapy, recreation therapy, habilitation therapy, and others.

The following case vignette illustrates several principles of psychopharmacotherapy with individuals with dementia, discussed below.

LG is an 88-year-old widowed primary care physician, a resident in an upscale nursing home, in reasonably good health for his age. Over a period of weeks, LG developed confusion, uncertainty, and depression. One evening, he "sundowned" into another male resident's room, whom he did not know well and with whom he did not have a previous relationship. He told the nurse who retrieved him from the other resident's room that he had been "distracted, that's why I went into Joe's room that night." LG had been on donepezil (Aricept®) for about three months, with stabilization of his prior forgetfulness. He was referred to the house physician assistant (PA).

The history that the PA obtained from LG and his daughter included several depressive episodes on LG's part in the 30 years since his wife's death, some treated with tricyclic anti-depressants, some not, and all associated, directly or indirectly, with grief and sadness for the loss of his wife. His daughter's impression was that LG generally responded well to anti-depressant psychopharmacotherapy. The PA started LG on a clinical trial of mirtazapine (Remeron®). Over the next several weeks, LG's mood cleared as did his periods of confusion and forgetfulness. In formal counseling sessions with a staff nurse ("…who reminds me of my daughter…") also helped LG maintain his mood and daily functioning. He attributed his clinical improvement, in part, to his "…sleeping better with the Remeron®. Thank you, doctor…"

This case vignette illustrates (1) The need to make one change at a time when multiple psychotropic agents are used. In this case, LG's donepezil (Aricept®) was maintained with the mirtazapine (Remeron®), leading to the impression that LG's clinical improvement was due, at least in part, to his sedating anti-depressant (i.e., mirtazapine; Remeron®). This further leads to the impression that (2) LG's forgetfulness was actually a symptom of pseudodementia (depressive symptoms presenting as dementia, especially in the elderly) and not the worsening of a dementing process. The vignette also illustrates (3) The need to take a full history. LG himself was not cognitively capable of giving the history to the house PA that his daughter could. That history, in turn, prompted the PA to think of pseudodementia in the differential diagnosis of LG's condition, and to prescribe mirtazapine (Remeron®). The diagnosis turned out to be correct, and the psychopharmacotherapy to be helpful.

Anti-feeding/eating Agents

As the "flip side" of "Anti-appetite Agents," this present class of psychopharmacotherapeutic agents serves as an adjunct to the primary modality of psychotherapy/counseling and behavioral approaches, with which individuals with eating/feeding disorders are treated. The *DSM-5* currently recognizes several types of feeding and eating disorders, as presented in Table 4.12.

As a practical matter, as presently practiced, psychopharmacotherapy has a limited role in the treatment of these disorders. As of this writing, fluoxetine (Prozac®) has FDA approval for treatment of bulimia nervosa, and lisdexamfetamine (Vyvanse®) for the treatment of binge eating disorder (BED). Other classes of anti-depressants, such as other SSRIs, MAOIs, and tricyclic anti-depressants have been used off-label, especially when depression is a "target" symptom. Olanzepine (Zyprexa®) and other atypical anti-psychotic medications appear beneficial for weight gain in anorexia nervosa, again through off-label use.

Considering the numerous organ systems adversely affected by eating disorders, especially anorexia nervosa, careful attention must be paid to assessing and treating the consequences of these disorders. This attention may be in conjunction with the primary non-medical treating professional (e.g., psychologist, social worker, counselor) if that is the treatment model, or alone, if the medical professional is the primary treating professional.

Table 4.12 Feeding and eating disorders per *DSM-5*

Pica
Rumination disorder
Avoidant/restrictive food intake disorder
Anorexia nervosa
Bulimia nervosa
Binge-eating disorder (BED)
Other specified feeding or eating disorder
Unspecified feeding or eating disorder

Anti-impotence Agents

For this subclass of "Anti-agents" in this *Primer*, it is useful to divide "impotence," or sexual dysfunctions, broadly speaking, into (1) *Primary* erectile dysfunction or hypofunction in men and low sexual drive (or, when meeting *DSM-5* Diagnostic Criteria, hypoactive sexual desire disorder, or HSDD) in women, *not* resulting from other causes, such as medication (including many psychotropic agents), medical conditions, and the like; (2) *Secondary*, resulting from other causes (as in "secondary to…"); and (3) *Combined* or mixed causes. Table 4.13 lists some secondary causes of sexual dysfunction.

Table 4.13 Secondary causes of sexual dysfunction

Type of cause	Examples
Psychiatric disorders	Anxiety disorders Dementia Depressive disorders Schizophrenia and other psychotic disorders
Psychotropic medications	Anti-cholinergic agents (see Chap. 2) Anti-depressant agents Anti-psychotic agents Barbiturates
Non-psychotropic medications	Anti-androgens (e.g., for cancer chemotherapy) Anti-hypertensive agents (especially centrally acting ones) Finasteride (Proscar®; others)
Drugs of abuse	Alcohol (licit, but abusable; see Chap. 5) Marijuana Opioids Stimulants/psychostimulants
Medical conditions	Acromegaly Addison's disease Diabetes Hyperthyroidism Hypothyroidism Klinefelter's syndrome (XXY genotype) Multiple sclerosis Parkinson's disease Pelvic surgery Pelvic irradiation Peripheral vascular disease (PVD) Spinal cord injury (SCI) Syphilis (Ives) Temporal lobe epilepsy (TLE)

Adapted from Black and Andreasen (2014)

Until the 1990s, the mainstay of treatment for sexual dysfunction was counseling/psychotherapy of a variety of types including cognitive behavior therapy (or CBT; see Chaps. 7 and 8) and the behaviorally oriented Masters and Johnson couples approach (using exercises such as "sensate focus" to heighten couple's sexual awareness); as well as counseling/psychotherapy, from the 1960s and 1970s.

In 1998, however, a vasodilator (PGE inhibitor) named sildenafil (Viagra®) received FDA approval for treating erectile dysfunction, and a new era of pharmacotherapy for sexual dysfunction began. Over the years, a raft of new agents for sexual dysfunction in men appeared and gained popularity. As recently as 2015, flibanserin (Addyi®) was FDA-approved for hypoactive sexual desire disorder (HSDD, per *DSM-5*) in premenopausal women. Table 4.14 presents these "anti-impotence" agents and their current clinical indications.

Table 4.14 Anti-impotence agents

Gender	Agent	Indications
Men	Alprostadil (Caverject®; others)	Erectile dysfunction
	Cyproheptadine (Periactin®; discontinued, generic only available)	No FDA indication; anorgasmia
	Sildenafil (Viagra®)	Erectile dysfunction
	Tadalafil (Cialis®)	Erectile dysfunction
	Testosterone (various preparations)	Hypogonadism
	Vardenafil (Levitra®)	Erectile dysfunction
	Vardenafil ODT (Staxyn®)	Erectile dysfunction
Women	Bremelanotide (Vyleesi®)	Hypoactive sexual desire disorder in premenopausal women
	Flibanserin (Addyi®)	Hypoactive sexual desire disorder in premenopausal women

Adapted from Puzantian and Carlat (2020)

Two additional agents, testosterone and cannabidiol (CBD), are worth mentioning. The former agent, testosterone, is available by prescription when clinically indicated, in a variety of types, preparations, and routes of administration. Clinical indications are hypogonadism and low serum testosterone; studies do not suggest clinical benefit in the presence of normal testosterone levels, notwithstanding media and other hype to the contrary.

Cannabidiol (CBD), available over-the-counter and in a variety of facilities, is a non-euphorigenic compound in marijuana, recently touted to be useful in pain management, anxiety and depression, sexual dysfunction, and a number of other conditions (see Chap. 5). Mechanisms proposed for the purported effectiveness of CBD in sexual dysfunction include a general relaxing and disinhibiting effect of sexual tension and performance anxiety, and a vasodilation effect in genital areas, not unlike the vasodilation of sildenafil (Viagra®) and other such medications. As of this writing, however, effectiveness of CBD in sexual dysfunction has not been demonstrated, to my knowledge, in formal studies (which, as a practical matter, are not required by the FDA for off-label use of medications and non-regulated products). The jury is still out on this question!

Last, for present purposes and focusing on medications and drugs (psychotropic, medical, and illicit) as potential causes of sexual dysfunction, the prescribing healthcare professional should approach individuals with sexual dysfunction as they would use a common-sense clinical approach: Take a careful and detailed history and drug history; include these several types of agents, when applicable, in a differential diagnosis of the basis, or cause, of the sexual dysfunction; and develop an investigation and treatment plan based, at least in part, on these data.

Anti-insomnia Agents

Even though sleep disorders are at least as prevalent in the community as anxiety, depression, bipolar disorder, and schizophrenia, their designation as a "Minor" Anti-agent in this particular book is simply because most pharmacologic intervention for insomnia, specifically, is not made by psychiatrists or other prescribing mental health professionals but rather by primary care practitioners.

Other sleep-wake disorders (i.e., in addition to insomnia) exist, which are classified in the *DSM-5* as what may be called "primary" sleep disorders (insomnia disorder, hypersomnolence disorder, excessive daytime sleepiness [EDS], and narcolepsy), i.e., sleep disorders per se; breathing-related sleep disorders (obstructive sleep apnea hypopnea, central sleep apnea, and sleep-related hypoventilation); circadian rhythm sleep-wake disorders; and parasomnias (characterized by abnormal behavior, physiological events, or odd experiences in association with sleep, sleep-wake transitions, or sleep architecture stages: "parasomnia," from the Greek, translates as the "opposite" of "sleep"). In this vein, sleep medicine is an enormous field, with pulmonologists, neurologists, and sleep medicine specialists. (Sleep medicine is a specific specialty recognized and monitored by the American Board of Medical Specialties, or ABMS.) Specialists are taking the lead in the care, treatment, and research of these disorders, with diagnostic sleep centers/laboratories widely available for polysomnographic sleep studies. Pharmacotherapeutic interventions are available for most of these sleep disorders and conditions.

For present purposes, this chapter focuses on pharmacotherapy of insomnia, the most prevalent (whether as a formal *DSM-5* disorder or a treatment symptom) of these sleep disorders, with "anti-insomnia agents," or "hypnotics."[2] For information, details, and pharmacotherapeutic recommendations concerning these other sleep disorders, the reader is referred to works cited in the Selected References in Chap. 1 of this *Primer*.

In recognizing the potential cause of insomnia for any given individual with that prevalent condition, the "primary" and "secondary" distinctions are a useful approach to treatment, psychopharmacotherapeutic or not.

> *First*, if an individual's insomnia is not caused by a specific diagnosable sleep disorder with a specific pharmacotherapeutic intervention, then "sleep hygiene" should be the start of any treatment plan. That term involves such practices as avoiding the use of stimulating substances such as tea, caffeinated coffee, spicy food, nicotine, alcohol (which can produce a stimulating withdrawal 6–8 hours after ingestion), exercise, and others, at bedtime; restricting bedtime to sleep (and sex) only, not to include extensive reading, computer work, strenuous exercise, and the like; regular exercise (but not strenuous exercise at bedtime), good diet and weight control; low light, comfortable sheets, and other such amenities to enhance the sleep environment; and relaxation exercises and behavioral interventions (such as CBT for insomnia, or CBT-I) before sleep.

---

[2] "Hypnotics," as opposed to "sedatives," the latter for inducing calmness during the day (see Chap. 3, section "Antianxiety Agents").

Second, if treatment of insomnia does call for psychopharmacotherapy, a wide variety of medications is available, with different pharmacologic properties (onset and duration of action, drug–drug and drug–food interactions, undesirable effects, and the like) from which to choose for individual patients/clients. These medications include some which have been discussed previously in this *Primer* and which are clinically indicated for other conditions, such as anxiety (i.e., the benzodiazepines: "Antianxiety Agents"). With the benzodiazepines, in particular, attention must be paid to abuse potential, as also discussed in Chap. 5.

Other potential side effects of concern with hypnotics—especially with the elderly—include development of tolerance with long-term use; withdrawal signs and symptoms with abrupt discontinuation; paradoxical (aggression, irritability) reactions to the agents; respiratory depression (especially for the elderly with the benzodiazepines); and benzodiazepines combined with opioids. With this last combination, a recent FDA "black box" warning concerned the serious and potentially fatal effects of that combination); anterograde amnesia (especially with the "z-drugs" and the benzodiazepines, and especially in the elderly); CNS depression; complex sleep-related behaviors (such as eating, driving, texting, and having sex, especially in combination with alcohol—a "black box" FDA warning about these behaviors with these agents was listed in 2019); and daytime sedation, hangovers, and grogginess.

Table 4.15 summarizes several medications and their classifications used as sedatives-hypnotics. (See also Chap. 3, section "Antianxiety Agents," for further information and details.)

Table 4.15 Anti-insomnia agents

Medication class	Examples	Comments
Anti-depressants (see Chap. 3, "Antidepressant Agents")	Doxepin (Silenor®; tricyclic anti-depressant) Trazodone (Desyrel®; Oleptro®) Mirtazapine (Remeron®; serotonin norepinephrine agonist)	Off-label for insomnia, except Silenor® Off-label for insomnia; discontinued, available as generic
Anti-psychotic (see Chap. 3, "Antipsychotic Agents")	Quetiapine (Seroquel®; in low doses)	Off-label for insomnia
Antihistamines	Diphenhydramin (Benadryl®; others)	Can cause confusion, especially in the elderly Doxylamine (Unisom®; others)
Benzodiazepines	Clonazepam (Klonopin®; brand discontinued, available as generic) Flurazepam (Dalmane®; brand discontinued, available as generic) Lorazepam (Ativan®; FDA-approved for GAD; off-label for insomnia) Temazepam (Restoril®; for short-term use) Triazolam (Halcion®; for short-term use)	Benzodiazepines as a group differ among one another in terms of pharmacologic properties such as rapidity of onset, half-life, duration of action, and the like. Some are FDA-approved for daytime use (sedative) and some are for nighttime use for sleep induction ("hypnotic")
Melatonin agonist	Ramelteon (Rozerem®)	
Dual orexin receptor antagonist	Suvorexant (Belsom*r*a®)	
"Z-drugs"	Eszopiclone (Lunesta®) Zaleplon (Sonata®) Zolpidem (Ambien®; others) Zolpidem low dose (Intermezzo®)	GABAergic action, like benzodiazepines, but lower sedation and addiction potential, reportedly

Adapted from Puzantian and Carlat (2020)

Anti-obsessive-compulsive Agents

Like a number of other psychiatric disorders for which psychopharmacotherapy may be indicated, no specific medication for this condition presently exists because the condition itself is not considered a discrete entity with a known neurobiological cause for which a specific and discrete psychopharmacologic agent would provide the "key" to the "lock" of the condition. As discussed early on in this *Primer*, this disorder's pathophysiologic mechanism of action ("cause") does not "carve nature at her joints."

In that context, the new chapter in the *DSM-5* entitled "Obsessive-Compulsive and Related Disorders" discusses obsessive-compulsive disorder (OCD) and other such conditions as being within an obsessive-compulsive spectrum. Table 4.16 lists these disorders as presented in the *DSM-5*.

Obsessive-compulsive disorders and its related conditions can be devastating in their effects on affected individuals. Treatment often consists of a behavioral psychotherapeutic approach (e.g., systematic desensitization, flooding; see Chaps. 7 and 8) in combination with a pharmacologic agent. For the latter, clomipramine (Anafranil®, an older tricyclic anti-depressant agent) and several SSRIs—all anti-depressant agents—have FDA approval for treatment of OCD. Other SSRIs are periodically used off-label for this indication. Table 4.17 summarizes these points.

Table 4.16 Obsessive-compulsive and related disorders per *DSM-5*

Obsessive-compulsive disorder (OCD)
Body dysmorphic disorder (BDD)
Hoarding disorder
Trichotillomania (hair-pulling disorder)
Excoriation (skin-picking) disorder
Substance/medication-induced obsessive-compulsive and related disorder
Obsessive-compulsive and related disorder due to another medical condition
Other specified obsessive-compulsive and related disorder
Unspecified obsessive-compulsive and related disorder

Table 4.17 Anti-obsessive-compulsive disorder (OCD) agents

Medication class	Examples	Comments
Anti-depressants: tricyclic antidepressant	Clomipramine (Anafranil®)	FDA indication for OCD
Anti-depressants: selective serotonin receptor inhibitors (SSRIs)	Fluoxetine (Prozac®; others)	FDA indication for OCD
	Fluvoxamine (Luvox®)	FDA indication for OCD
	Fluvoxamine ER (Luvox CR®)	FDA indication for OCD
	Paroxetine (Paxil®; others)	FDA indication for OCD
	Paroxetine CR (Paxil CR®)	FDA indication for OCD
	Sertraline (Zoloft®; others)	Off-label for OCD
Anti-depressants: serotonin norepinephrine reuptake inhibitors (SNRIs)	Desvenlafaxine (Pristiq®)	Off-label for OCD
	Venlafaxine (Effexor®)	Off-label for OCD

The following case vignette illustrates "classic" OCD in an individual whose life trajectory was characteristic of this disorder, and whose treatment was unremarkable, and—fortunately—helpful.

JZ is a 28-year-old former accounting student, living for the past two years with his girlfriend, working as a bookkeeper with a small manufacturing company, and an individual who had always taken pride in his meticulous and careful work. Over about a six-month period, he became increasingly careful and rigid in his personal and professional life, engaging in taking long showers and washing his hands as often as he could, and in frequently checking and rechecking light switches, faucets, moving furniture to right-angle positions, and in other such compulsive behaviors. These compulsions reached the point at which JZ's girlfriend at first suggested, and then insisted, that he consult a healthcare professional for help.

JZ consulted a psychiatric APN (advanced practice nurse), who referred him to a local psychologist, who in turn treated him with a CBT-desensitization program. This program seemed to help for a few weeks. However, after that, JZ's symptoms and signs increased to the point that he felt paralyzed at work, and unable to do much at home except for shower, wash his hands, and check light switches. He re-consulted the APN, who prescribed fluoxetine (Prozac®), initially 20 mg. in the morning. Over several months, the APN increased his dose to 80 mg. and continued to follow him as an outpatient. JZ's signs/symptoms remitted gradually over several months, and he was able to return to a reasonable approximation of his earlier life.

Over the years, JZ remained stable and productive with his combined therapy, maintaining his fluoxetine (Prozac®) on an ongoing basis, with periodic "refreshers" of his CBT-desensitization therapy with the psychologist. Periodically, JZ and his APN attempted to reduce his dose of Prozac®, invariably resulting in a return or exacerbation of his OCD symptomatology.

Eventually, JZ accepted that he would be on Prozac® "for a long time," and no longer questioned his treatment plan. By then, he and his girlfriend had married and had a child. JZ managed the additional stresses of these major life changes well, without an exacerbation of his OCD symptomatology.

This vignette illustrates several features of the ongoing treatment of OCD including the need to rule out possible underlying medical causes or influences on JZ's OCD condition, the effectiveness of combined modalities of therapy with his condition, the need to maintain both modalities of treatment in this chronic condition, the need to maintain high doses of fluoxetine (Prozac®), and the need for communication and coordination among treating professionals.

Anti-pain Agents

Also known as "analgesics," this group of medications is extensive, covering a wide variety of types and classes of medications, and a focus of clinical attention in a burgeoning clinical specialty called "pain management," or "pain medicine."

Along with anxiety, depression, and insomnia, pain is one of the most reported and most treated symptoms in clinical practice.

The definition of pain per the IASP (International Association for the Study of Pain) Task Force on Taxonomy is "An unpleasant sensory and emotional experience associated with actual or potential tissue damage, or described in terms of such damage" (Merskey H, Bogduk N, editors. Part III: Pain terms. A current list with definitions and notes on usage. In: Classification of chronic pain. 2nd ed. IASP Press; 1994. p. 209–214.)

And in his writings of 1914, Dr. Albert Schweitzer vividly described pain in these words: "Pain is a more terrible lord of mankind than even death itself" (Schweitzer A. On the edge of the primeval forest. The Macmillan Company; 1931).

A full review of pain management is well beyond the scope of this present section, and the reader is referred to any number of books, articles, electronic databases and directories, internet sources, and the like for information and details about this vast topic.

For present purposes, it is useful to categorize pain condition and pain psychopharmacotherapy in several discrete ways, as presented in Table 4.18. Each of these categories will be discussed, in turn, in the rest of this chapter.

"Acute" vs. "chronic" pain refers to pain that lasts for fewer than 30 days or more than 30 days, respectively. Conceptually, acute pain syndromes are generally easier for healthcare practitioners to understand, empathize with, and treat, since analgesia, by definition, is achieved relatively quickly. Difficult and elaborating behavioral/psychiatric symptomatology is generally not present or minimally present with these patients/clients. "Chronic" pain, on the other hand, refers to pain syndromes that last more than 30 days, are often difficult for the healthcare practitioner to understand, empathize with, and treat, and generally include significant behavioral/psychiatric overlay. A variety of chronic pain syndromes has been identified and characterized in the pain management field, depending on the origin and pathophysiology (e.g., ischemic cardiovascular and peripheral neurologic pathology, and others), the cause (e.g., neoplasm), location, and other such parameters.

In this vein, chronic malignant pain (CMP, resulting from on underlying neoplastic process) vs. chronic benign pain (CBP, not resulting from an underlying neoplastic process) is a useful contrast, in that an important approach to both of these types of patients/clients is to diagnose and treat the underlying causative condition, whatever it might be, to the extent possible. The longstanding controversy in this area about the advisability of prescribing long-term opioid medications for chronic benign pain has gone through cycles and phases, in this writer's experience, over the years. In the 1980s, chronic opioid use was considered ill-advised because of concerns about tolerance, overdose, the therapeutic index, and potential danger of opioids especially when taken with other agents, and death, either inadvertently or on purpose. As with hallucinogens (psychedelics), healthcare professionals prescribed these agents conservatively and sparingly (see also, Chap. 4 concerning hallucinogens/psychedelic agents).

However, in the 1990s and the early 2000s, with the advent of "pain as the fifth vital sign" (an approach and campaign which has since been discontinued), the more liberal use of opioid psychopharmacotherapy was seen as a swing of the prescribing pendulum, and the prescribing of opioids for benign chronic pain syndromes became more acceptable in the healthcare community.

Then, with the onset and worsening of what has been referred to variously as the current "opioid epidemic," or "opioid crisis" in the early 2010s, the pendulum of opioid prescribing practices has swung back to conservative approaches, and more careful scheduling and tracking of opioids and related compounds (e.g., Federal and State "Prescription Drug Monitoring Programs," or PDMPs). A number of different factors has been considered responsible for the uptick of licit and illicit opioids and related drugs and drug-related deaths during this time frame, including the far-reaching effects of the "pain as a fifth vital sign" movement, the ready availability of potent opioids (such as Fentanyl® and Carfentanyl®), the sense in the general population that licit and illicit drugs can resolve problems in living, and so forth. These points will be discussed further in Chap. 5.

"Central" vs. "peripheral" pain refers to the cause and pathophysiology of different pain syndromes. "Central" pain syndromes refer to those that arise in the CNS itself (recognizing that any pain sensation can be modulated, elaborated, or modified by higher centers of the brain, since pain is, at its core, a neurologic phenomenon) or are modified by CNS influences. "Peripheral" pain syndromes, in contrast, refer to those that originate in somatic tissue damage and are medicated through afferent nervous pathways to central brain areas. The concept of using psychotropic agents (in contrast to strictly analgesic agents), such as anti-convulsants (see above), to influence and modify pain perception is based on this distinction. The following two tables (Tables 4.18, and 4.19) further illustrate these points.

Finally, for present purposes, the dichotomous distinctions in pain syndromes presented in Table 4.18 are actually the same, the first ("real" vs. "imagined" pain) couched in the common-sense terminology often perceived by individuals who work with real-world patients/clients in pain, and the second couched in more technical terminology. As a practical matter, whether pain is "real" or "not real" is a

Table 4.18 Categories of pain conditions for purposes of this *Primer*	Acute (nociceptive) vs. chronic pain
	Chronic benign pain (CBP) vs. chronic malignant pain (CMP)
	Central vs. peripheral pain
	"Real" vs. "imagined" pain
	Pain without significant psychiatric contribution vs. pain with significant psychiatric contribution (somatic symptom disorder)

Table 4.19 Variants and terms for chronic pain

Nociceptive (somatic) pain	Neuropathic pain
Syrinx formation (central cavitation)	Chronic nerve syndrome
Causalgia	Central dysesthesia syndrome
Central pain	Allodynia
Phantom limb pain	Hyperpathia
Dysesthesia	Neural injury pain

Adapted from Velez D. *CME program* (2008)

meaningless distinction, since as a subjective symptom, "pain"—whether plausible to the onlooker or not—is "real" to the person in pain, and in the healthcare context, needs to be addressed in some way by the evaluating and/or treating healthcare professional.

From a psychiatric viewpoint and, from the diagnostic perspective, pain syndromes which are more elaborated and less straightforward than short-term acute situations (which would be less likely to require psychiatric/psychological/counseling intervention than more complex symptomatology) are specifically embodied in the *DSM-5* as "Somatic Symptom and Related Disorders," depicted in Table 4.20. Although the current edition of the *DSM* no longer endorses what may be termed "elaborated" pain disorder, this broad category of disorders includes pain syndromes, emphasizing an individual's response to pain and/or other symptoms rather than to the pain symptoms themselves.

Focusing on psychopharmacotherapeutic agents, the following "World Health Organization Analgesic Ladder" outlines four steps in terms of increasing potency of medications and interventions involved in the evaluation and treatment of different pain syndromes.

Table 4.20 Somatic symptom and related disorders, per *DSM-5*

Somatic symptom disorder
Illness anxiety disorder
Conversion disorder
Psychological factors affecting other medical conditions
Factitious disorder imposed on self and imposed on another
Other specified somatic symptom and related disorder
Unspecified somatic symptom and related disorder

For examples of analgesic medications, their doses and dosing schedules, and other such information about the various non-steroid anti-inflammatory drugs (NSAIDs), opioids, non-opioids, and other agents in this table, the reader is referred to applicable textbooks, monographs, internet services, electronic databases, and the like.

For purposes of this chapter, several specific psychotropic medications for two specific syndromes, peripheral neuropathic pain syndromes and fibromyalgia—both with significant psychiatric components—will be reviewed next.

First, concerning peripheral neuropathic pain syndromes, two psychotropic medications of two different classes—duloxetine (Cymbalta®), an anti-depressant, and pregabalin (Lyrica®), a novel anti-convulsant—have FDA-indications and off-label uses in these areas. Duloxetine (Cymbalta®) is approved for diabetic peripheral neuropathic pain, fibromyalgia, and other chronic musculoskeletal pain syndromes (and other off-label chronic pain disorders). Pregabalin (Lyrica®) is approved for diabetic peripheral neuropathic pain, neuropathic pain associated with spinal cord injury, postherpetic neuralgia, and fibromyalgia (and other non-pain indications, including partial complex seizures, generalized anxiety disorder, and withdrawal from benzodiazepines and alcohol; these last three are off-label uses).

Second, fibromyalgia as a chronic pain condition is characterized by widespread and chronic pain, fatigue, and cognitive impairment ("fibro fog"). For proper diagnosis, the presence of some of the 18 "tender points" designated by the American College of Rheumatology, first in the 1990s, is no longer required. A number of co-morbid or co-occurring conditions may be seen with fibromyalgia, including irritable bowel syndrome, migraine and other types of headaches, interstitial cystitis or painful bowel syndrome, temporomandibular joint (TMJ) disorder/dysfunction, and others. These frequent comorbidities confer a strong psychiatric component to this condition. The psychopharmacotherapy of fibromyalgia rests on three principles: (1) Use of non-opioid analgesic agents as depicted in the "World Health Organization Analgesic Ladder" (Table 4.21) for amelioration and relief of pain not complicated by psychiatric symptomatology or overlay; (2) Use of an FDA-approved agent specifically for fibromyalgia, once the diagnosis is made and confirmed, namely duloxetine (Cymbalta®), pregabalin (Lyrica®), or milnacipran (Savella®, a serotonin-norepinephrine reuptake inhibitor, or SNRI), or other such off-label agent with which the prescriber is familiar and experienced; and (3) Use of other psychopharmacotherapeutic agents to address the fibromyalgia patient's psychiatric "target symptoms."

No discussion of "Anti-pain Agents" would be complete without some mention of headaches and headache pain. Without going into the details and nuances of the types, classifications, diagnostic approaches, treatment, and the like about headaches and headache pain, and without underestimating the prevalence and

Table 4.21 World Health Organization analgesic ladder	
Step 4: Invasive and minimally invasive treatments
Step 3: Opioids from moderate to severe pain ± non-opioid agents ± adjuvants
Step 2: Opioids from mild to moderate pain + non-opioid agents ± adjuvants
Step 1: Non-opioids ± adjuvants
Adapted from Anekar A, Castella M. *WHO analgesic ladder* (2020)

significance of headaches as a public health concern, the rest of this section will focus on the psychopharmacotherapy of migraine and cluster headaches. As a practical matter, a variety of analgesic and psychotropic medications have been used for migraine prophylaxis (prevention) and for aborting migraine attacks. Table 4.22 lists such medications, non-psychotropic and psychotropic. As with other sections of this chapter, for further information and details about migraine and other headache pathophysiology, diagnosis, treatment, doses and dose scheduling, and the like, the reader is referred to applicable textbooks, monographs, articles, internet sources, electronic databases, and the like.

Although this section has focused on psychopharmacotherapy of different types and syndromes of pain conditions, the beneficial role of psychotherapy/counseling, behavioral intervention, weight control, exercise, and other such

Table 4.22 Medications for migraine prevention and treatment

Class	Examples (P) = prophylaxis (A) = abort attacks	Indications
Non-psychotropic agents	Non-steroidal anti-inflammatory drugs (NSAIDs) (A)	Acetaminophen (Tylenol®; others) Naproxen (Aleve®; others) Aspirin Ibuprofen (Advil®; others)
	Stimulants (A)	Caffeine/ergotamine (Migergot®; others)
	Triptans (A)	Sumatriptan (Imitrex®; others)
	Antihistamines (A)	Diphenhydramine (Benadryl®; others)
	Beta-blockers (P)	Metoprolol (ToprolXL®; others)
	Calcium channel blockers (P)	Verapamil (Isoptin®; others)
	ACE inhibitors (P)	Lisinopril (Prinivil®; others)
Psychotropic agents	Tricyclic anti-depressants (P)	Amitriptyline (Elavil®; others)
	Novel anti-convulsants (P)	Topiramate (Topamax®; others); Gabapentin (Neurontin®)
	Anti-convulsants (P)	Valproic acid (Depakote®; others)
	Selective serotonin reuptake inhibitors (SSRIs) (P)	Fluoxetine (Prozac®; others)

non-pharmacologic interventions should not be underestimated for these conditions. Such interventions are discussed in Chaps. 6, 7, and 8 in this book.

Last, to illustrate some of the dilemmas encountered in frequent clinical scenario-treating chronic benign pain syndromes with opioid pharmacotherapy on a long-term basis, the following case vignettes present examples, respectively, of a "good" candidate and a "bad" candidate for long-term opioid pain management therapy. These vignettes incorporate a number of biopsychosocial features in their evaluations. Both individuals were seen for consultation/evaluation in an acute general community hospital by the hospital's Consultation-Liaison Psychiatry Service.

WO, a 43-year-old married female insurance executive from the suburbs, wife of an attorney and mother of two older teenage children, was involved in a motor vehicle accident in which she sustained a T10 fracture dislocation. This injury rendered WO paraplegic with an inconsistent sensory level between T8 and T10. WO had been a happy and productive wife, mother, and professional, who had exercised and played tennis regularly throughout the year, and who has no past personal or family history of psychiatric disorder or substance abuse.

Seriously depressed and angered initially by her accident and her paraplegia, WO gradually came to accept her condition to some extent after several months of inpatient and day hospital rehabilitation, physical therapy and psychotherapy/counseling alone and with her husband. She did not require potent analgesic medication during that time.

However, after several weeks, WO developed the rapid onset of dysesthesia, burning, and occasionally lancinating low-back pain. This pain increased and persisted over several weeks. WO's initial pharmacologic treatment consisted of increasing non-narcotic analgesic medication (prescribed on a maintenance basis), with the addition of Elavil (25 mg. at hour of sleep) to this regimen. WO's response to these changes in her treatment plan was inconsistent. Psychiatric consultation was requested to evaluate WO for a trial of chronic long-term opioid therapy.

CK is a 20-year-old male, who at age 10, while playing across the street from his house, sustained a gunshot wound to his back. This injury left CK paraplegic, wheelchair- and bed-bound, with an inconsistent sensory level between T8 and T0, where T10 was the site of impact of the bullet in CK's gunshot wound.

CK was electively admitted to the hospital for surgical correction of a back ulcer. CK had a known and long history—both before and after his back trauma—of polysubstance abuse and addiction. For this reason and to assist in CK's medical management, the Consultation-Liaison Psychiatry Service was consulted by CK's treatment team.

At the age of 16, CK required the placement of surgical rods in his back in order to correct a progressive kyphosis. These rods were removed approximately 2½ years later, and an abscess formed in the area of removal several months after that. CK developed a full-blown decubitus which had not healed by the time of his elective admission, and which became very large as a result of multiple infections. These infections required hospitalizations for antibiotic therapy and debridement, and CK was noted during those hospitalization to have been a management problem and demanding of analgesic medications (primarily opioids).

CK had been inactive at home for a number of years, despite a large and supportive family. He had been treated with multiple pain medications at home, and he also acknowledged using four to five Percodan® tablets every three hours, as well as two 5 mg. Valium® every four to six hours, above and beyond the non-narcotic analgesic medications prescribed for him by his family physician on a maintenance basis. In addition to his prescription drug supplementation with Percodan®, CK also supplemented his medication regimen with alcohol, marijuana, and illicit acetaminophen (Tylenol®) with codeine.

CK underwent myocutaneous and paraspinal flap closure of the decubitus during this elective hospitalization. At the time that the Psychiatry Service was consulted for CK, his prescribed medication regimen was Percocet® (two tablets every three hours as needed) and Valium (5 mg. every six hours as needed) with Clinitron® therapy. CK's nurses noted his difficult and demanding behaviors, especially around his analgesic regimen. CK complained that the prescribed medications (i.e., Percocet® and Valium®) were not holding him for the full three hours for which they were prescribed.

Therefore, Consultation-Liaison Psychiatry was consulted for advice in managing and medicating (pain medication) CK, particularly with regard to the evaluation of CK for a trial of long-term (maintenance) opioid therapy.

Anti-panic Agents

Of anxiety disorders, broadly speaking, ongoing manifest panicky symptoms, in general, may be considered as bursts of intense anxiety, tension, and other symptoms on an unpredictable or random basis ("panic attacks") or in a recurrent pattern over time ("panic disorder"). In that vein, the *DSM-5* distinguishes between those two conditions, emphasizing the multi-organ system symptomatology (e.g., the "*DSM-5* Panic Attack Specifier" gives a number of such symptoms, including palpitations, diaphoresis, tremulousness, chest pain, choking sensation, dizziness, numbness and tingling, nausea and abdominal distress, and others) of panic attacks and panic disorder.

As with the anxiety disorders in general and many other psychiatric disorders, the optimal approach to the treatment of panic disorder is multidisciplinary, including psychotherapy/counseling, psychopharmacotherapy, combination approaches (especially cognitive behavior therapy [CBT] and psychopharmacotherapy), life style modification, diet and weight control, exercise, avoidance of stimulants/psychostimulants, and the like. Focusing on psychopharmacotherapy, for present purposes, the mainstay psychopharmacotherapeutic agents for panic disorder are the benzodiazepines (specifically alprazolam [Xanax®; others], clonazepam [Klonopin®; others], with others used off-label) and anti-depressants (SSRIs: fluoxetine [Prozac®; others], paroxetine [Paxil®; others], and sertraline [Zoloft®; others], with others used off-label). Venlafaxine ER (Effexor XR®) is also FDA-approved for panic disorder, and desvenlafaxine (Pristiq®; others) is used off-label for the same indication. As an off-label use for what may be considered a forme fruste of a panic attack, propranolol (Inderal®; others) is given for performance anxiety ("stage fright") and akathisia (motor restlessness; see Chap. 3, section "Antipsychotic Agents"), especially for individuals with marked somatic symptomatology as part of their anxiety or panic. These uses are in addition to the FDA-approved indications of propranolol (Inderal®; others) for hypertension, atrial fibrillation, migraine prophylaxis, postmyocardial infarction cardioprotection, and essential tremor.

The reader is cross-referenced to those sections of "Antianxiety Agents" and "Antidepressant Agents" concerning benzodiazepines and SSRIs/SNRIs for further information and details about these psychopharmacotherapeutic agents. The second case vignette (AB) for "Antianxiety Agents," for example, illustrates an individual with panic disorder.

Antiparkinsonian Agents

As discussed in the Preface of this volume, psychiatry as a medical specialty and a relative newcomer into medicine was almost interchangeable during the latter half of the nineteenth century: Neurologists took care of chronic patients in "insane asylums" (what are now called state or county mental hospitals); psychiatrists in office practices evaluated and treated patients with such neurologic conditions as conversion disorders, or paralyses ("hysterical neurosis"); and vice-versa, with interchange among these physicians. As both fields evolved over the years, they diverged, with neurologists taking care of individuals with cerebrovascular accidents (CVAs or "strokes"), degenerative disorders, neoplastic disorders, seizures, and the other panoply of conditions which are now called neurologic disorders. Psychiatry diverged toward psychological constructs and inferences about which are now called psychiatric disorders.[3] In about the 1960s, however, as medical technology and psychopharmacology grew and became more sophisticated, the evidenced-based foundations of both fields began to drive them back together, giving definition to areas of training and practice such as neuropsychiatry and behavioral neurology.

One area of practice and research which is a good example of this convergence of the disciplines of neurology and psychiatry is Parkinson's disorder. This degenerative multisymptomatic disorder was identified in 1817 by the English neurologist, Dr. James Parkinson, after whom the disorder was named, and who himself called the condition "paralysis agitans." Dr. Parkinson's original description of the condition, and his subsequent study and treatment over many years, focused on the motoric aspects of the condition, namely the "Parkinsonian tremor, bradykinesia, poverty of motion, mask-like facies," and so forth.

More recently, however, the interest and focus of neurology and psychiatry in Parkinson's disease have been on three major areas of symptomatology often manifested by Parkinsonian patients, viz., (1) motoric, (2) behavioral, and (3) neuropsychiatric/cognitive. All of the foregoing is to say that the treatment of individuals with Parkinson's disease is of increasing interest and practice to psychiatrists, especially concerning behavioral and neuropsychiatric symptomatology associated with the disease.

---

[3] For an engaging account of these two branches of medicine during the American "Gilded Age," with a forensic bent, see Rosenberg CE. *The trial of the assassin Guiteau: psychiatry and the law in the gilded age*. University of Chicago Press; 1968.

In addition to Parkinson's disease as a focus of psychiatric interest, also of interest are the terms "Parkinsonian" and "Parkinsonism," descriptors for the types of dystonias (movement disorders) seen as a side effect in a number of psychotropic medications (especially first-generation anti-psychotic agents of the high-potency, low-dose type). This section will focus on both of these areas of interest.

In this area of Parkinson's disease—the neuropsychiatric/cognitive area—clinical depression (in as many as half of Parkinson's patients) and psychosis (with delusions and hallucinations) are not uncommon. For psychopharmacotherapy of the former (depression), a wide range and variety of anti-depressants are available to treat these co-occurring "target symptoms," although care must be taken not to use agents significantly affecting dopaminergic neurotransmitter systems. Dopamine agonist medications which directly address the dopamine deficiency of Parkinson's disease must necessarily be in careful balance with other agents affecting the dopamine system. For psychopharmacotherapy of the latter (psychosis), the prescriber also has to be careful about the balance between dopamine-blocking properties of most anti-psychotic agents (see "Anti-psychotic Agents" in this chapter) and dopamine depletion in Parkinson's disease. As of this writing, only one anti-psychotic agent, pimavanserin (Nuplazid®)—the only non-dopamine blocking atypical anti-psychotic currently available—has FDA approval specifically for psychosis in Parkinson's disease, although the recency and expense of this agent are of concern. In this context, as a practical matter, quetiapine (Seroquel®) has been used frequently for Parkinson's disease, as well as for treating insomnia, both as off-label use.

Parkinsonism, also known as extra-pyramidal syndrome, or EPS, refers to several medication-induced movement disorders, or dystonias, caused by a variety of medications—both psychopharmacologic and non-psychopharmacologic—primarily, for present purposes, the conventional/traditional ("first-generation") high-potency, low-dose anti-psychotic agents, such as haloperidol (Haldol®) and fluphenazine (Prolixin®). These dystonias consist of a Parkinsonian tremor at rest, rigidity, akathisia, akinesia, (late-onset) tardive dyskinesia (TD), cogwheeling, bradykinesia, and mask-like facies. Pharmacologic treatment of EPS focuses on anticholinergic agents (see Chap. 2, section "Three Additional Classes"), with others and cardiac drugs also useful. Table 4.23 presents these agents.

Table 4.23 Antiparkinsonian agents

Drug class	Examples	Comments
Anti-cholinergic/ antimuscarinic compounds	Benztropine (Cogentin®; others) Biperiden (Akineton®; others) Diphenhydramine (Benadryl®; others)	Antihistamine with anti-cholinergic preparations
	Ethopropazine (Parsidol®; others)	Phenothiazine derivative with anti-cholinergic preparations
	Orphenadrine (Norflex®; others)	Muscle relaxant (CNS)
	Pramipexole (Mirapex®; others) Procyclidine (Kemedrin®; others) Trihexyphenidyl (Artane®; others)	Also indicated for restless leg syndrome
Dopamine facilitators	Amantadine (Symmetrel®; others) Entacapone (Comtan®; others)	Used as adjunct in Parkinson's disease
Beta-blockers	Beta-propranolol (Inderal®; others)	Antihypertensive agent; monitor BP carefully
Alpha-agonists	Clonidine (Catapres®; others)	Antihypertensive agent; monitor BP carefully. (See also section "Anti-addiction Agents" in this chapter and Chap. 5)

Recognizing tardive dyskinesia as a Parkinsonian movement disorder, until relatively recently, no specific pharmacologic agent was available for this condition. Treatment involved dosage scheduling of the causative medications (usually anti-psychotic agents), changing the anti-psychotic medications, drug holidays, and the like. However, three specific medications have recently become available to treat tardive dyskinesia (and in the case of tetrabenazine [Xenazine®] to treat the choreiform dystonias of Huntington's disease), viz., valbenazine (Ingrezza®), deutetrabenazine (Austedo®), and tetrabenazine (Xenazine®). Other agents used secondarily for the treatment of tardive dyskinesia include amantadine (Symmetrel®), benzodiazepines, and the OTC and health food agents gingko biloba extract and vitamin E. Tardive dyskinesia, again, is a common side effect of high-potency, low-dose conventional/traditional, "first-generation" anti-psychotic agents, but can also result from long-term and chronic use of dopamine-blocking agents for other indications, such as the antiemetic metoclopramide (Reglan®) and prochlorperazine (Compazine®). Adventitious movements characteristic of tardive dyskinesia include chewing, grimacing, tongue protrusion, lip smacking, and other repetitive, writhing, oro-bucco-lingual facial movements.

Anti-pseudobulbar Affect Agents

The extreme mood swings and uncontrollable affect known as "pseudobulbar affect" is another example (see section "Antiparkinsonian Agents" in this chapter) of the convergence of psychiatry and neurology as disciplines over the past 40–50 years. This neuropsychiatric condition is part of the symptom complex in "pseudobulbar palsy," an upper motor neuron lesion caused by bilateral disturbances of the corticobulbar track resulting from vascular, degenerative, neoplastic, and other such etiologies involving cranial nerves IX, X, and XII. This condition is characterized by motor signs, such as impairment in, or inability to control, facial and related movements (such as speaking, dysphagia, smiling, chewing, grimacing, and others) and emotional signs and symptoms of labile affect, and uncontrollable fits of laughter and crying (the portrayal of the main character, Arthur Fleck, in the 2019 movie, *Joker*, is a good illustration of this condition). Bulbar palsy is a lower motor neuron lesion involving the same cranial nerves with the same motor deficits, but without the marked affective lability and symptomatology of pseudobulbar palsy.

Although pseudobulbar palsy was first identified and characterized in the 1800s, specific pharmacotherapy for this condition did not come into being until 2010, with FDA-approval of a combined preparation of dextromethorphan and quinidine called Nuedexta®. As of this writing, Nuedexta® is the only FDA-approved drug for that particular indication, although it has also been used off-label for individuals with Parkinson's disease and dementia. Conversely, off-label use of a variety of anti-depressant agents, and cognitive therapy, has also been approaches to the treatment of pseudobulbar affect.

Anti-sex Agents

Conceptually, the opposite of "Anti-impotence Agents" are "Anti-sex Agents," intended to influence, control, and reduce what may be called "hyper-sexed" behaviors of such individuals as paraphilics, pedophiles, and sex offenders. Like many of the other "Anti" categories of medications presented and discussed in this *Primer*, this "Anti" category is not a distinct category per se but rather consists of other psychotropic agents, especially SSRI anti-depressants.

The field of paraphilic (from the Greek: "para" meaning "opposite," and "philia" meaning "love") disorder has a long and notorious history, including historical figures such as the Marquis de Sade (the term "sadism" derives from his name), Richard F. von Krafft-Ebbing (who, in 1886, wrote *Psychopathia Sexualis*), Henry Havelock Ellis (who co-authored *Sexual Inversion*, originally published in 1896), and others, and covers a variety of anomalous sexual activity preferences and deviant patterns of sexual arousal, behaviors, interests, and activities. Paraphilia (abnormal and deviant sexual interests and behaviors) and paraphilic disorders (patterns of abnormal and deviant sexual interests, behaviors, and thoughts leading to a formal diagnosis) are given in Table 4.24; a full discussion of these topics is well beyond the scope of this *Primer*.

For present purposes, the general approach to treatment of individuals with para-philias includes behavioral/counseling/psychotherapeutic (especially cognitive behavior therapy or CBT, with specialized approaches in sex-offender-specific treatment or SOST, for example), with psychopharmacotherapy. The latter includes two broad pharmacotherapeutic classes of agents, viz., hormonal agents (for more severely symptomatic individuals, generally) and psychotropic agents (for less severely symptomatic individuals, generally). Each of these two categories may be further divided into two sub-categories, as displayed in Table 4.25.

Table 4.24 Paraphilic disorders per *DSM-5*

Voyeuristic disorder
Exhibitionistic disorder
Frotteuristic disorder
Sexual masochism disorder
Sexual sadism disorder
Pedophile disorder
Fetishistic disorder
Transvestic disorder
Other specified paraphilic disorder
Unspecified paraphilic disorder

Table 4.25 Anti-sex agents

I. *Hormonal agents* (antiandrogenic effects)
    A. Indirect-acting mechanisms of action
        1. Progestin analogue (feminizing hormone)
           Medroxyprogesterone (Depo-Provera®; others)
        2. Gonadotrophin hormone-releasing hormone (GrRH) agonists/Luteinizing hormone-releasing (LHRH) agonists
           Leuprolide acetate (Lupron®; others), depot preparations
           Leuprorelin (Lucrin®; others)
           Goserelin acetate (Zoladex®; others)
           Triptorelin (Triptodur®; Trelstar Depot®; others)
    B. Direct-acting mechanisms of action (androgen receptor blockade)
        1. Cyproterone acetate
        2. Flutamide (Eulexin® Oral; others)
        3. Finasteride (Propecia®; others)

II. *Psychotropic agents*
    A. Agents for treatment of male aggressive hypersexuality (mainstay: SSRI anti-depressant agents)
    B. Agents for treatment of co-occurring (comorbid) psychiatric symptoms (target symptoms) and conditions
    C. Specific off-label applications
        Naltrexone (Revia®; others)
        Methylphenidate (Ritalin®; others)

Adapted from Greenfield D. *Journal of Psychiatry Law* (2006)

Currently, even though surgical intervention is not a prevalent current treatment modality, for completeness' sake, mention will be made of this modality. Essentially, two surgical approaches to hypersexuality have been practiced, the first for many years. These approaches are (1) surgical castration (orchiectomy, a practice going back at least to the Middle Ages, if not earlier) and (2) stereotactic brain surgery (not used in the United States). While studies indicate that these approaches are effective in reducing sex drive and sex offending recidivism, the irreversibility of the procedures and the medico-legal and ethical concerns have made these approaches little used in current practice. The following case vignette illustrates some of these concerns and issues:

> EH is a 37-year-old male patient/client in maintenance SOST (sex offender specific treatment), court-ordered, with a serious sex offense history in his late teenage years. He has been on court-ordered community supervision as a "Megan's Registrant" since his release from incarceration ten years ago for his earlier sex offenses.
>
> Until about a year ago, EH had been doing well clinically—without recurrent sexual acting out—on two sequential SSRI anti-depressant agents, regular individual and group SOST. EH has a well-paying and steady job, a casual relationship with a male friend "from when I was a kid," and an active-enough social life with friends and family.
>
> After a difficult spell at work about a year ago, EH began to feel strong and uncomfortable sexual urges and cravings. Psychological intervention and support from his SOST staff, and several different psychopharmacotherapeutic changes, including a course of anti-androgenic medications, still left him feeling desperate and worried about his status as a registrant with his "Megan's" community notification program.
>
> Finally, he spoke with both his SOST psychologist and his prescribing Physician Assistant, requesting referral to an urologist "who would be willing to castrate me." Initial inquiries were unsuccessful.

As mentioned above, a full discussion of even only the psychopharmacotherapy of this fascinating and troubling field of "hyper-sexed" individuals, paraphilics, and sex offenders is well beyond the scope of this chapter. The field is replete with psychiatric, neuropsychiatric, medical, biochemical, pharmacologic, legal, ethical, criminological, and societal controversies, as well as other such issues and concerns, some raised by the case vignette just presented. For further discussion about these disorders and their treatment, the reader is referred to the *DSM-5* and to other applicable books, monographs, electronic databases, articles, internet sources, and the like.

Anti-trauma Agents

The last of the sixteen "Minor Anti-agents" in this classification system are those used to treat symptomatology of trauma, especially of post-traumatic stress disorder (PTSD) and acute stress disorder (ASD), as articulated in the *DSM-5*. Like many of the disorders and syndromes discussed in Chaps. 3 and 4, specific traumatic manifestational symptomatology corresponding exactly to traumatic stimuli, or stressors do not exist in nature. For that reason, and in view of the protean manifestations of traumatic symptomatology, several psychopharmacotherapeutic "Anti-agents" have been shown to be useful in ameliorating traumatic symptomatology, and several have FDA-approval for treating symptoms of PTSD. Specifically, several SSRIs—paroxetine (Paxil®; others), sertraline (Zoloft®; others), and fluvoxamine (LuvoxCR®)—have FDA-approval for PTSD; two SNRIs—venlafaxine (Effexor®) and desvenlafaxine (Pristiq®; others)—are used off-label for PTSD; and as a practical matter, other SSRIs are probably indicated for PTSD as well, depending on patient/client characteristics (e.g., fluoxetine [Prozac®] for patients/clients without prominent sleep disturbances). However, considering the affect storm in PTSD and the "black box" FDA warning about suicidality with anti-depressants, these agents should be used conservatively and carefully monitored.

In addition, prazosin (Minipress®, an anti-depressant agent) is often used to treat PTSD victims with nightmares, as an off-label indication.

Several benzodiazepines (e.g., clonazepam [Klonopin®; others] and diazepam [Valium®; others]) are used off-label to reduce PTSD-associated anxiety but should be restricted to short-term use, owing to abuse potential, especially in individuals with histories of chemical dependency.

In the final analysis, as recognized by the U.S. Department of Veterans Affairs, among others, the first-line treatment for PTSD ought to be psychological (counseling; psychotherapy). Cognitive-behavioral therapy (CBT), eye movement desensitization and refocusing (EMDR), and controlled exposure desensitization, are among the effective behaviorally oriented therapy modalities (see Chaps. 7 and 8) for these conditions, and individual supportive counseling/psychotherapy, family, and group psychotherapy are among such effective non-behavioral therapy modalities.

Historically, the concept of what the *DSMs* (since *DSM-III*, in 1980) have called post-traumatic stress disorder, or PTSD, has gone back hundreds, perhaps thousands, of years. "DaCosta's syndrome" and "soldier's heart," (both terms from the American Civil War era), "shell shock" (World War I era), "battle fatigue" (World War II era), "post-traumatic neurosis" (in earlier *DSMs*), and other terms have been used to describe this prevalent and serious condition.

A full review of this vast and complex condition is well beyond the scope of this section of this *Primer*, which has focused on an overview of a secondary approach to the treatment of this condition, namely psychopharmacotherapy. For further information and details about PTSD and other traumatic conditions, the reader is referred to applicable textbooks, the *DSM-5*, monographs, electronic databases, internet sources, and other such sources, including those given in the Selected References for this volume.

A Note on References

Rather than burdening the reader with excessive and detailed references and citations in this *Primer*, given below are particularly useful selected references. In addition, other specific references and citations will be given in parentheses throughout the *Primer*. For further information and details about any topics presented and discussed in this book, the interested reader is referred not only to the following list of selected references, but also to applicable textbooks, monographs, electronic databases, print articles and materials, internet sources, and other applicable resources.

Selected References

- Black DW, Andreasen NC. Introductory textbook of psychiatry. 6th ed. American Psychiatric Publishing, Inc.; 2014. (A solid basic textbook of psychiatry.)
- Multiple Authors. Diagnostic and statistical manual of mental health disorders (*DSM-5*). 5th ed. American Psychiatry Association, Inc.; 2013. (This book is the controversial "bible" for primarily American and Canadian psychiatric diagnoses.)
- The comparable international work to the *DSM-5* is currently the 2019 International classification of diseases (*ICD-10*). 10th ed. World Health Organization. (The *ICD-11* was due for adoption in 2020.)
- Frances A. Saving normal: an insider's revolt against out-of-control psychiatric diagnosis, big pharma, and the medicalization of ordinary life. Harper Collins Publishers; 2013. (The subtitle says it all! See Chap. 4 in this *Primer*.)
- Ghaemi SN. Clinical psychopharmacology: principles and practice. Oxford University Press; 2019. (A scholarly, detailed, and lengthy overview of psychopharmacology, also covering social practice and research/methodologic aspects of the field.)
- Hales RE, Yudofsky ST, Roberts LW, editors, et al. The American Psychiatric Publishing textbook of psychiatry. 6th ed. American Psychiatric Publishing, Inc.; 2014. (A standard, detailed encyclopedic textbook tome, for reference. A seventh edition is available, copyright 2019, with updated coverage in a number of areas.)
- Harrington A. Mind fixers: psychiatry's troubled search for the biology of mental illness. W.W. Norton and Company; 2019. (A historical and scholarly review of the topic, including some of the same topics as *Saving Normal* listed above.)
- Puzantian T, Carlat DJ. Medication fact book for psychiatric practice. 6th ed. Carlat Publishing, LLC; 2020. (A very useful "cookbook" for psychotropic prescribing, conveniently organized and presented for the practitioner.)
- Watters E. Crazy like us: the globalization of the American psyche. Free Press; 2010. (Psychiatric diagnostic issues similar to those in *Saving Normal*, with an international focus.)
- Weil A. Mind over meds: know when drugs are necessary, when alternatives are better—and when to let your body heal on its own. Little, Brown and Company; 2017. (A balanced and holistic approach to pharmacology and psychopharmacology by the popular "guru" of these fields.)

Selected Internet References

With the surfeit of internet resources, websites of all imaginable types and quality, and numerous related electronic sources of information and data, the reader, clinician, researcher, and member of the public—patient/client or not—may easily become confused about where to go and what to accept in learning psychopharmacology and psychopharmacotherapy. In this vein, a productive way to navigate the bewildering array of such sources consists of dividing them into several categories, viz.

1. Refereed ("peer-reviewed;" "juried") scientific, technical, and professional journals, newsletters, and the like, including e-journals, e-newsletters, and other open-source e-publications. Selected examples include:

   - *Journal of Clinical Psychopharmacology* (peer-reviewed independent professional journal)
   - *Experimental & Clinical Psychopharmacology* (peer-reviewed professional journal of the American Psychological Association)
   - *Journal of Psychopharmacology* (peer-reviewed professional journal of the British Association for Psychopharmacology)
   - *Psychopharmacology* (Berlin/Heidelberg; Springer Publications)

2. Government and academic/research institutions, publications and e-publications, and associated websites. Selected examples include:

   - National Institute of Mental Health (NIMH) website, affiliated institutes, programs, centers, websites, and publications (electronic and print)
   - National Institute on Alcoholism and Alcohol Abuse (NIAAA) website, affiliated institutes, programs and centers, and websites and publications (electronic and print)
   - National Institute on Drug Abuse (NIDA) website, affiliated institutes, centers, programs and websites, and publications (electronic and print)
   - Canadian Centre on Substance Abuse (CCSA), affiliated programs and publications (electronic and print)
   - National Center on Addiction and Substance Abuse at Columbia University (NCASACU), programs and publications (electronic and print)

3. Journals, magazines, societies, and associated websites. Selected examples include:

   - *Psychology Today*
   - *Scientific American*
   - *Scientific American Mind*

As a practical matter, in researching particular topics electronically in psycho-pharmacology/psychopharmacotherapy, the logical rule—as with everything else—is to search for topic(s), keyword(s), and the like on a search engine, then to narrow the search with entries given by the search engine. An important factor to keep in mind here is the reliability, accuracy, and quality of the source: Sources from (1) and (2)—above—are considered more reliable than those in (3), generally. Those in (3), in turn, are generally considered more reliable than personal blogs, newsletters, product websites, company websites, and the like.

Chapter 5
Illicit Substances and Drugs

The field of substance abuse, chemical dependency, drug and alcohol abuse, and other such designations—all to be used interchangeably in this *Primer*—is a vast one, for which a full and comprehensive review is well beyond the scope of this volume. For that, the reader is referred to the Selected References at the end of the Preface of this *Primer* and, as before, to applicable electronic databases, internet sources, and the like.

Referring to Chap. 2 ("Basic Principles of Pharmacology, Psychopharmacology, and Psychopharmacotherapy") in this *Primer* and for purposes of this chapter, psychotropic agents may be categorized in several ways:

1. One such way is in terms of the various psychiatric disorders, conditions, and symptoms for which the agent is used in treatment. The four "Major Anti-s" and the sixteen "Minor Anti-s" are examples of this system of categorizing these agents.
2. Another way is in terms of whether use of the agents is licit (legal) or illicit (illegal). These categories recognize considerable overlap among agents, in that virtually any legitimate psychotropic agent—or any non-psychotropic agent, for that matter—may be misused or abused. Conversely, some usually illicit drugs may have licit indications, depending on their legal status (medical marijuana is a good recent example of this).
3. "Lumpers" and "Splitters." Lumpers: In terms of taxonomies, these individuals seek to create broad categories or taxons of things, collecting multiple characteristics and examples into few taxons. Splitters: In contrast, these individuals seek to create narrow categories, or taxons of things, collecting narrow and few characteristics and examples into many taxons. In the chemical dependency context, Lumpers generally distinguish in terms of the broad psychoactive effects of these drugs, for example: among stimulants, or psychostimulants; depressants; and hallucinogens, or psychotomimetics. Examples are presented in Table 5.1.

D. P. Greenfield, *Psychopharmacology for Nonpsychiatrists*, https://doi.org/10.1007/978-3-030-82507-2_5

4. From an applied clinical perspective, a fourth way of categorizing the addictions generally—i.e., not only those involving drugs and alcohol—is in terms of chemical and behavioral addictions. Table 5.2 lists some of both.
5. With respect to addiction medicine, a youthful distinction is made between medications which treat the chemical addictions per se (known as "medication-assisted treatment," or MAT) and those that treat symptomatology ("target symptoms") of addicts and alcoholics. Table 5.3 summarizes these points.

In this chapter, the distinction between "licit" and "illicit" substances, between chemical and behavioral addictions, and between MAT and psychopharmacotherapeutic treatment of symptoms of various addictive conditions will be presented and discussed. *DSM-5* treatment of what are termed in the *DSM-5* as "Substance Use Disorders" (SUDs) will also be covered.

The conclusion of this chapter will review non-pharmacologic approaches to the treatment of addicts and alcoholics, emphasizing the strong need for multidisciplinary and "continuum of care" treatment of these often difficult and challenging patients/clients.

Table 5.1 "Lumper" and "splitter" taxonomies of drugs

	Drug class	Examples (L = Licit; I = Illicit)
Lumpers	**Stimulants/psychostimulants** (see also "anti-ADHD agents;" and "anti-appetite agents") **Depressants** (see also "antidepressants") **Hallucinogens** (psychotomimetic)	Cocaine (L & I) Amphetamines/methamphetamines (L & I) Caffeine (L) Methylphenidate compounds (L & I) Many others Alcohol (L) Opioids (L & I) Barbiturates (L) Benzodiazepines (L & I) and "Z-drugs" (L) Many others Lysergic acid diethylamide (LSD) (I) Phencyclidine (PCP) (I) Cannabis sativa (marijuana) (L & I) Psilocybin (I) Ayahuasca (L & I) Synthetic marijuana (I) Khat (I) Ketamine ("special K;" Spravato®) (L & I)
Splitters	Alcohol, caffeine, cannabis (including synthetic marijuana), "designer drugs," hallucinogens, inhalants, opioids, sedatives/hypnotics/anxiolytics, stimulants, others or unknown	

Table 5.2 Chemical and behavioral addictions

Nature of addiction	Examples
Chemical addictions	Alcohol Caffeine Cannabis (marijuana) Hallucinogens/psychotomimetic Inhalants Opioids Sedative – hypnotics Stimulants/psychostimulants Tobacco
Behavioral addictions	Exercise Food (obesity) Gambling (listed in the *DSM-5*) Internet gaming Internet surfing Kleptomania Love Sex Shopping Tanning Texting/emailing Work ("workaholism")

Table 5.3 Medication-assisted treatment (MAT) and symptomatic treatment of addicts and alcoholics

I. **Agents That Treat Chemical Addictions Per Se**
Medication-assisted treatments (MATs):
For opioid addiction (OUD)
Methadone
Naltrexone (IR and L-A [Vivitrol®, Injectable])
Buprenorphine (Subutex®; Suboxone® [buprenorphine]) and other preparations
Naloxone (for emergency opioid overdose)
Clonidine (Catapres®)
Lofexidine (Lucemyra®)
For alcohol addiction (AUD)
Disulfiram (Antabuse®)
Acamposate (Campral®)
Naltrexone (Revia®)
For smoking (tobacco products) addiction
Nicotine replacement therapy (patches, polacrilex gum, others); "vaping" replacement therapy
Varenicicline (Chantix®)
Bupropion (Zyban®, for smoking specifically)
II. **Agents That Treat Symptomatology of Addicts and Alcoholics**
(See Table 2.5 in Chap. 2, "The Twenty Licit Anti-Agents")

Controlled Dangerous Substances (CDS)

In 1970, the Controlled Substance Act (CSA) of the FDA created a series of five categories of "dangerous drugs" on a sliding scale of five "Schedules" (I–V) from those considered the most dangerous (Schedule I) to those considered the least dangerous in terms of safety and abuse potential. These prescriptions were monitored by the (then) Bureau of Narcotics and Dangerous Drugs (BNDDs), later called the Drug Enforcement Administration (DEA) of the Department of Justice of the United States government. Review of the agents in these several categories in Table 5.4 indicates that while some agents are strictly "illicit" (i.e., CDS Schedule I) with "no accepted medical use," most—and most of the medications and agents discussed in this *Primer*—can be both, depending on the circumstances under which they are prescribed, whether prescribers follow acceptable federal and state guidelines (this can be especially problematic in the case of medical marijuana, in which in a number of states this prescribing is legal under proper conditions, but in which the federal jurisdiction, marijuana[1] remains illicit), and other such circumstances. For these reasons, it behooves the health professional registered and authorized to prescribe CDSs, "Scheduled Drugs," or "Controlled Substances" (the terms are used interchangeably here) to know and to stay abreast of (1) the CDS law and regulations in the state or other jurisdiction in which they practice and (2) the procedures and processes of the Prescription Drug Monitoring Program (PDMP), which provides electronic searchable databases for tracking licit CDS patients and their prescriptions, in the state or other jurisdiction in which they practice. The former can be searched in the annual update of *Title 21 Code of Federal Regulations* (www.fda. gov/medical-devices/medical-device-databases/code-federal-regulations-title-21-food-and-drugs) and the latter in the website for the PDMP Training and Technical Assistance Center (www.pdmpassist.org).

---

[1] <Footnote ID="Fn1"><Para ID="Par15">A word about "CBD" (cannabidiol) is pertinent here. Cannabidiol is a phytocannabinoid plant product related to **<Emphasis aid:cstyle="Bold" Type="Bold">cannabis sativa</Emphasis>**, the psychoactive and psychotomimetic compound in marijuana and hashish. Cannabidiol is one of many such related compounds and does not itself have psychoactive effects on consumers; is not a prescription-only medication or a Controlled Dangerous Substance; and is widely available in pharmacies, health food stores, and through the internet. It is touted as beneficial for a multitude of health conditions, including pain syndromes, tension and anxiety, general malaise, anorexia, and bulimia, and others, reportedly without dependency potential or deleterious psychiatric symptomatology. This <Emphasis Type="Italic">*Primer*</Emphasis> does not take a position on the usefulness (or not) of CBD, but it does note the widespread and burgeoning popularity of this cannabinoid and recommends further searching and researching on the part of the interested reader.</Para></Footnote>

Table 5.4 The controlled dangerous substances (CDS) schedules

CDS schedule	Characterization	Prescribing patterns	Examples
I	No accepted medical use, high potential for abuse, illegal to possess or use	May not be prescribed at all (with the exception of medical marijuana in some states)	Heroin, LSD, ecstasy, and others Marijuana (though legalized in some states, it is still illegal at the federal level)
II	High potential for abuse, but legal for medical use	May be prescribed only 1 month at a time, cannot be refilled, may not be called in, and patient must give the pharmacy a paper script (unless using an e-prescribing program that is DEA-certified, and that allows prescribing of controlled substances)	All psychostimulants, such as amphetamine and methylphenidate Opiates that are especially potent, such as oxycodone, fentanyl, and others Vicodin® (hydrocodone and acetaminophen) was recently rescheduled from Schedule III to Schedule II
III	Lower potential for abuse than Schedule I or II, but still quite abusable	May be refilled up to 5 times (no more than 6 months); may be called in	Suboxone® (buprenorphine/naloxone) Ketamine Xyrem® (sodium oxybate) Anabolic steroids Barbiturates Dronabinol (Marinol®)
IV	Lower potential for abuse than Schedule III	May be refilled up to 5 times (no more than 6 months); may be called in	All benzodiazepines (e.g., clonazepam, lorazepam, etc.) Various hypnotics, such as zolpidem, zaleplon, and suvorexant (Belsomra®) Wake-promoting agents, like modafinil and armodafinil Tramadol (Ultram®) Carisoprodol (Soma®) Lorcaserin (Belviq®), an anti-obesity drug
V	Lowest potential for abuse	May be refilled as many times as prescriber chooses (e.g., for 1 year or more); may be called in	Pregabalin (Lyrica®) Cough preparations with small amounts of codeine such as Robitussin AC® Antidiarrheal (Lomotil®; diphenoxylate/atropine)

Adapted from Puzantian and Carlat (2020)

DSM-5 **Considerations**

Concerning *DSM-5* and other characterizations of the licit and illicit chemical dependencies, Table 5.5 presents the core clinical features of the category of psychiatric disorders which the *DSM-5* calls "Substance Use Disorders," or SUDs. Going beyond the features and diagnostic criteria for SUDs in the *DSM-5*, Table 5.6 gives factors affecting an individual's response to a given drug. These factors recognize that such responses are determined by more than the drug, or agent itself: In effect, these factors are an application of the Epidemiologic Triangle model discussed in Chap. 1.

Table 5.5 *DSM-5* features of substance use disorders (SUDs)

"A problematic pattern of substance use leading to clinically significant impairment or distress, as manifested by at least TWO symptoms occurring within a 12-MONTH PERIOD…"
Social impairment
Impaired control
Risky use
Neuroadaptive/withdrawal
Mild, moderate, severe (symptoms); course specific (duration)

Table 5.6 Factors affecting an individual's responses to a drug

Pharmacology of the drug
Mental set of the drug user
Setting of the drug use
Biological vulnerability of the user
Route of administration of the drug (PO; IM; IV; IN; SC; etc.)
Co-occurring (comorbid) conditions and symptomatology of the user

Adapted from NIDA (1980s)

Chemical and Behavioral Addictions

Another area of addiction medicine, or addictionology, is in the relatively recent recognition of the non-chemical addictions, or behavioral addictions. Table 5.2 gives examples of such addictions or dependencies. In this broadened view of addictions, it is significant that the only non-chemical dependency listed in the *DSM-5* is "Gambling Disorder." Without doubt, other behavioral disorders will be given in further iterations of the *DSM*. From a psychologic perspective, a common mechanism of the various addictions is in the strong actions of the dopaminergic reward system in addicts, which increases the repetitive and reinforced nature of their neurologic activity along with a reduction in what translates clinically as good judgment and an increase in what translates clinically as denial: "I can stop/quit any time" and "The other guy'll get hooked, not me." This neurobiological commonality between the chemical and behavioral addictions is a basis, in part, for the next topic in this chapter, viz., Medication-assisted treatment (MAT).

Medication-assisted Treatment (MAT)

While psychopharmacotherapy is not the only approach to the treatment of addicts and alcoholics, in one type of addiction—opioid addiction—in particular, "medication-assisted treatment" or MAT (Table 5.3) has been shown during the recent and ongoing opioid crisis[2] to be a real life saver! Data and studies from the federal agencies, Centers for Disease Control and Prevention (CDC) and the National Institute on Drug Abuse (NIDA), demonstrate the effectiveness of MAT in preventing deaths from opioid overdose and in clinically helping to stabilize addicted individuals. As Table 5.3 shows, however, MAT can also be used in other chemical dependencies. The actual agents used in MAT derive from several "Anti-Agents" already discussed, including Anti-pain Agents (opioid antagonists, "blockers"), antihypertensives, and Antidepressant Agents. Since addicts and alcoholics often present with myriad physical and psychiatric symptoms, and with co-occurring (comorbid) psychiatric disorders, they will often request and/or need psychotropic medications drawn from such "Anti-Agent" classes as antidepressants, antianxiety agents (especially benzodiazepines), anti-manic agents, anti-insomnia agents, and others. And since the genesis of many of addicts' and alcoholics' problems and symptoms is generally from the agents that they request in those circumstances, the free and willy-nilly prescribing of such psychotropic agents for those patients/

---

[2] <Footnote ID="Fn2"><Para ID="Par22">While a detailed discussion of what has been called the current "Great Opioid Crisis" is well beyond the scope of this book, the excessive prescribing, diversion, and use of both licit and illicit opioids, resulting in dramatic overdose mortality from 2014 to the present, has been identified as one of most serious social and public health crises in the 2000s, on a par with the COVID-19 pandemic.</Para></Footnote>

clients is not indicated. These are individuals who have to learn to cope with life's stressors without chemicals (i.e., psychopharmacotherapeutic agents), for the most part, not with them. Striking a balance between MAT and other psychopharmaco-therapy comprises both the art and science of treating addicts and alcoholics.

Treatment Settings for the Addictions: A Continuum of Care

This last point brings up the issue of the treatment setting for addicts and alcoholics. Such settings range from outpatient counseling with a non-mental health professional (e.g., teacher, friend, priest, etc.) to medical inpatient services, with intermediate settings between those two poles, along with what is called a "continuum of care" model. The *ASAM* (*American Society of Addiction Medicine*) *Criteria* presents a good conceptual model of this continuum. (See Table 5.7, as adapted from the *ASAM Criteria*.)

A full discussion of treatment settings for the addictions, like other topics in this book, is well beyond its scope. A particularly good reference for this topic, and many others in this field, is the multi-authored (2018) *ASAM Principles of Addiction Medicine, Sixth Edition* to which the reader is referred, along with electronic databases, other books and articles, and internet sources, for further information and details.

Table 5.7 Continuum of care in addiction treatment

Stage of intervention	Type of intervention/treatment
1 (least intense)	None
2	Early intervention
3	Outpatient treatment (counseling, psychotherapy)
4	Intensive outpatient program (IOP) Partial hospital program (PHP)
5	Residential/inpatient programs Low-intensity residential High-intensity residential
6 (most intense)	Medically managed intensive inpatient program, including detoxification services

Adapted from the *ASAM Criteria* (2015)

Psychedelics

Spurred on to some extent by best-selling author Michael Pollan's *How to Change Your Mind: What the New Science of Psychedelics Teaches Us About Consciousness, Dying, Addiction, Depression and Transcendence* (Pollan 2018) and after having lain dormant from the 1960s until the early 2000s, clinical research and treatment with psychedelic (classified for present purposes as "hallucinogens") agents has become a hot new topic in psychiatry, addiction medicine, psychology and counseling, and other areas of health care.

The history of these compounds goes back to prehistoric times, when such psychedelic agents as psilocybin, peyote, and ayahuasca were used in rituals and shamanistic practices by many pretechnological societies. Systematic scientific interest and study of these agents may be traced to "Bicycle Day" (April 19, 1938), when Dr. Albert Hoffman, a Swiss industrial chemist, ingested microdoses of lysergic acid diethylamide (LSD) in his research laboratory, rode his bicycle, and experienced the first documented psychedelic "trip" (it was a vivid and good one!). Research and scientific, clinical, and sociologic interest in hallucinogens and psychedelics grew over the next decades, accelerated in part by a seminal *Life* magazine article in 1957 called "Seeking the Magic Mushroom" until the 1960s.

During the turbulent 1960s, counterculture "bad trips," the ill-fated Harvard Psilocybin Project of Dr. Timothy Leary and Dr. Richard Alpert, and the 1970 Controlled Substances Act (which placed LSD, PCP, marijuana, psilocybin, and other hallucinogens and psychedelics into CDS Schedule I—which is still the case; see Table 5.4—effectively making them illegal) all soured society and the scientific community on psychedelics and led to a dearth of study, research, and optimism about the possible role of these compounds for human well-being. An abbreviated history of these events and others is presented in Table 5.8.

In 2006, a banner year for psychedelic research into clinical application, several significant events occurred, marking the modern renaissance of psychedelic research. These events are presented in Table 5.9.

As a result of these and later events and trends, scientific, societal, and clinical interest has grown dramatically in these and other related compounds over the past two decades, with no end in sight. Perhaps the advent of, at first, legalized medical marijuana in many states, and legalized recreational marijuana in fewer but a growing number of states, are manifestations of this interest and trend. Psilocybin, in particular, is the core of clinical research at two major medical centers in the United States: Johns Hopkins Center for Psychedelic & Consciousness Research and NYU Langone Health, among others. Studies are underway in the application of psychedelics ("mind-dissolving" agents also known as "entheogens," or "generating the divine within")—purportedly without the abuse potential of illicit agents, if used properly—for applications in the study and treatment of anxiety, trauma, depression, addiction, consciousness, and the mental and emotional stresses of death and dying.

Psychedelics are back!

Table 5.8 Events in the history of psychedelics

Era:	Events:
Pre-historic	**Psychedelic agents known to be used by pre-historic humans**: Psilocybin Peyote Ayahuasca Others: Rituals; shamanic practices
1938	**LSD discovered by Dr. Albert Hoffman on April 19, 1938** (henceforth known and celebrated as "Bicycle Day")
1950s	**Brain science:** "Soup v. Sparks" Neurotransmitters, clinical applications LSD (lysergic acid dimethylamine) Psilocybin ("teonanacatl" or "flesh of the gods" by the Aztecs) **Psychedelics were "good."**
1957	**Article appears in *Life* magazine: "Seeking the Magic Mushroom,"** by R. Gordon Wasson, May 13, 1957
1960s	**Counterculture "acid trips"** **Leary and Alpert** **"Turn on, tune in, drop out."** **Harvard Psilocybin Project** **Psychedelics were "bad."**
1970s & 1980s	**Controlled Substance Act, 1970**
1990s & 2000s	**Renaissance of:** Neuroscience Psychotherapy "Psychonauts" Treatment of: Anxiety – trauma Depression – dying Addiction – consciousness Organized studies: NYU Langone Health Johns Hopkins CPCR Others **Psychedelics are "back."**

Table 5.9 Three significant events for psychedelics

100th anniversary, in 2018, of the birth of Albert Hoffman, Ph.D., discoverer of LSD. ("Bicycle Day," April 19, is celebrated annually.)

Under the Religious Freedom Restoration Act of 1993, U.S. Supreme Court allowed the importing of ayahuasca, with DMT (CDS Schedule I) for sacramental purposes, by União do Vegetal (UDV), a Native American religious sect.

Seminal scientific paper "Psilocybin Can Occasion Mystical-Type Experiences Having Substantial and Sustained Personal Meaning and Spiritual Significance," by R. Griffiths et al. (2006). In *Psychopharmacology*. Springer Nature.

Evaluating and Treating Addicts and Alcoholics

No essay on illicit substances and drugs would be complete without some discussion of the "host" (in the Epidemiologic Triangle model)—the patient/client—in this context. In that vein, rather than presenting a case as such, Table 5.10 presents salient features and hallmarks of a paradigmatic drug-seeking patient/client. The interviewing/examining clinician needs to be aware of these potential "con-men/women" and able to deal with them in a calm, compassionate, but firm manner. It is not per se illegal to be duped, but it is illegal for a prescriber to continue prescribing to the scammer.

Table 5.10 Simulated interview: behaviors and hallmarks of the drug-seeking patient/client

1. New patient, new physician (new practice)
2. From a long distance away
3. Very well dressed
4. Late (in the day) visit, without a scheduled appointment
5. Immediately before a holiday weekend
6. Young (22–50 years old)
7. Requests specific analgesics only
8. Describes "classic" pain syndrome
9. Gives "textbook description" of a known disease
10. Behavior is quiet when nobody is looking
11. Behavior is agitated and painful when somebody is looking (the "Pain Show")
12. Lacks involuntary autonomic features associated with pain
13. Factitious ("faked") vital signs where possible
14. Referral patterns are vague and evasive (doesn't name the referring physician or give plausible reasons for the referral)
15. Ingratiating, unctuous approach to the physician ("I heard you really cared about patients with pain.")
16. Paranoid, guilt-provoking attitude toward the physician ("If you don't help me, you'll force me to get what I need on the street.")
17. Occupational history is vague and evasive
18. History of doctor-shopping and multiple hospitalizations (when history is obtainable)
19. Knows psychopharmacology, and CDS in particular, very well
20. Offers payment in cash for visit
21. Blaming and "conning" the physician
22. Insists on "drug of choice"
23. Refuses to submit blood or urine samples for toxicology screen (TDS)

A Note on References

Rather than burdening the reader with excessive and detailed references and citations in this *Primer*, given below are particularly useful selected references. In addition, other specific references and citations will be given in parentheses throughout the *Primer*. For further information and details about any topics presented and discussed in this book, the interested reader is referred not only to the following list of selected references but also to applicable textbooks, monographs, electronic databases, print articles and materials, internet sources, and other applicable resources.

Selected References

- Black DW, Andreasen NC. Introductory textbook of psychiatry. 6th ed. American Psychiatric Publishing, Inc.; 2014. (A solid basic textbook of psychiatry.)
- Multiple Authors. Diagnostic and statistical manual of mental health disorders (*DSM-5*). 5th ed. American Psychiatry Association, Inc.; 2013. (This book is the controversial "bible" for primarily American and Canadian psychiatric diagnoses.)
- The comparable international work to the *DSM-5* is currently the 2019 International Classification of Diseases (*ICD-10*). 10th ed. World Health Organization. (The *ICD-11* was due for adoption in 2020.)
- Frances A. Saving normal: an insider's revolt against out-of-control psychiatric diagnosis, big pharma, and the medicalization of ordinary life. Harper Collins Publishers: 2013. (The subtitle says it all! See Chap. 4 in this *Primer*.)
- Ghaemi SN. Clinical psychopharmacology: principles and practice. Oxford University Press: 2019. (A scholarly, detailed, and lengthy overview of psychopharmacology, also covering social practice and research/methodologic aspects of the field.)
- Hales RE, Yudofsky ST, Roberts LW, et al., editors. The American Psychiatric Publishing textbook of psychiatry. 6th ed. American Psychiatric Publishing, Inc.; 2014. (A standard, detailed encyclopedic textbook tome, for reference. A seventh edition is available, copyright 2019, with updated coverage in a number of areas.)
- Harrington A. Mind fixers: psychiatry's troubled search for the biology of mental illness. W.W. Norton and Company; 2019. (A historical and scholarly review of the topic, including some of the same topics as *Saving Normal* listed above.)
- Puzantian T, Carlat DJ. Medication fact book for psychiatric practice. 6th ed. Carlat Publishing, LLC; 2020. (A very useful "cookbook" for psychotropic prescribing, conveniently organized and presented for the practitioner.)
- Watters E. Crazy like us: the globalization of the American psyche. Free Press; 2010. (Psychiatric diagnostic issues similar to those in *Saving Normal*, with an international focus.)

- Weil A. Mind over meds: know when drugs are necessary, when alternatives are better—and when to let your body heal on its own. Little, Brown and Company; 2017. (A balanced and holistic approach to pharmacology and psychopharmacology by the popular "guru" of these fields.)

Selected Internet References

With the surfeit of internet resources, websites of all imaginable types and quality, and numerous related electronic sources of information and data, the reader, clinician, researcher, and member of the public—patient/client or not—may easily become confused about where to go and what to accept in learning psychopharmacology and psychopharmacotherapy. In this vein, a productive way to navigate the bewildering array of such sources consists of dividing them into several categories, viz.

1. Refereed ("peer-reviewed;" "juried") scientific, technical, and professional journals, newsletters, and the like, including e-journals, e-newsletters, and other open-source e-publications. Selected examples include:

   - *Journal of Clinical Psychopharmacology* (peer-reviewed independent professional journal)
   - *Experimental & Clinical Psychopharmacology* (peer-reviewed professional journal of the American Psychological Association)
   - *Journal of Psychopharmacology* (peer-reviewed professional journal of the British Association for Psychopharmacology)
   - *Psychopharmacology* (Berlin/Heidelberg; Springer Publications)

2. Government and academic/research institutions, publications and e-publications, and associated websites. Selected examples include:

   - National Institute of Mental Health (NIMH) website, affiliated institutes, programs, centers, websites, and publications (electronic and print)
   - National Institute on Alcoholism and Alcohol Abuse (NIAAA) website, affiliated institutes, programs and centers, and websites and publications (electronic and print)
   - National Institute on Drug Abuse (NIDA) website, affiliated institutes, centers, programs and websites, and publications (electronic and print)
   - Canadian Centre on Substance Abuse (CCSA), affiliated programs and publications (electronic and print)
   - National Center on Addiction and Substance Abuse at Columbia University (NCASACU), programs, and publications (electronic and print)

3. Journals, magazines, societies, and associated websites. Selected examples include:

- *Psychology Today*
- *Scientific American*
- *Scientific American Mind*

As a practical matter, in researching particular topics electronically in psycho-pharmacology/ psychopharmacotherapy, the logical rule—as with everything else—is to search for topic(s), keyword(s), and the like on a search engine, then to narrow the search with entries given by the search engine. An important factor to keep in mind here is the reliability, accuracy, and quality of the source: Sources from (1) and (2)—above—are considered more reliable than those in (3), generally. Those in (3), in turn, are generally considered more reliable than personal blogs, newsletters, product websites, company websites, and the like.

Chapter 6
Botanicals, Herbals, Nutraceuticals, and (Dietary) Supplements ("Natural Products")

This heterogeneous grouping of non-prescription agents called "Botanicals, Herbals, Nutraceuticals, and (Dietary) Supplements," or BHNSs, for present purposes does not "fit" easily into biochemically and pharmacologically based categories: Their commonality, for purposes of this *Primer*, is that they are widely available (pharmacies, supermarkets, health food stores, and others); have a broad range of therapeutic and adverse effects; are very popular; are part of current prevalent trends in holistic and personal healthcare lifestyles, and education (complementary and alternative medicine, or CAM; diet and exercise[1]; and the like); are almost all available over-the-counter (OTC; see Chap. 2); are often a source of patients'/clients' questions for their healthcare providers; and are of increasing interest to mental health professionals and other healthcare providers for psychopharmacotherapeutic reasons. These compounds are generally not regulated by the FDA, leaving the consumer faced with uncertain claims by the manufacturers, and the categories of these compounds and products overlap considerably, leaving some confusion about what they are and what they do.

For all of these reasons, it behooves the prescribing professional to have at least a rudimentary understanding of the nature, scope, and applications of these agents. The purpose and intent of this chapter are to provide such an understanding.

Table 6.1 gives a broad overview of the areas of treatment in the field of Complementary and Alternative Medicine (CAM), including more than botanicals, herbals, nutraceuticals, and supplements. CAM is also a vast topic well beyond the scope of this *Primer*; the reader is referred, in particular to: Micozzi M, editor. Fundamentals of complementary, alternative, and integrative medicine. 6th ed. Elsevier, Inc.; 2019 for both broad overviews and encyclopedic in-depth coverage of this field, as well as to other texts and monographs, electronic databases, internet sources, and the like.

---

[1] My dentist, a very holistic and preventive practitioner herself, has told me for years that with "…diet, exercise, tooth flossing, and not smoking, you'll live forever…".

© The Author(s), under exclusive license to Springer Nature
Switzerland AG 2022
D. P. Greenfield, *Psychopharmacology for Nonpsychiatrists*,
https://doi.org/10.1007/978-3-030-82507-2_6

Table 6.1 Topics in holistic health and complementary and alternative medicine (CAM)

Aromatherapy	Manual therapies and bodywork
Chiropractic	Massage
Diet and weight control	Meditation and mindfulness practices
Essential oil therapy	Naturopathy and naturopathic medicine
Exercise (for depression and cognitive decline)	Clinical nutrition
Herbal medicines	Osteopathic manipulative techniques
Hydration	(OMT)
Light therapy (for seasonal affective disorder, or SAD; see Chaps. 3 and 9)	Yoga and other forms of mind/bodywork

Since many products in the fields of holistic health and CAM are not regulated by the FDA or other health-related oversight agencies, questions may arise of dose equivalents, bioavailability of active ingredients, standardization among brands, adulterants among products, and other such concerns in what may be termed "quality control" of these very varied products. So, as a practical matter—as with making choices among a wide variety of psychotropic agents for the same clinical indication—the most sensible practice, in my view, is for patients/clients and their consulting healthcare professionals to become familiar with a narrow group of specific non-regulated agents and then stay with that particular agent and brand (e.g., St. John's wort, for depression).

Focusing on the four entities presented in this chapter, Table 6.2 gives definitions, examples, and uses of these entities.

Table 6.2 Botanicals, herbals, nutraceuticals, and (dietary) supplements, including overlapping products and applications

Topic	Definition	Examples	Applications
Botanicals	Plant products used as additives	Gin (juniper berry), anise, arugula extract, orris root, lemon peel, baobab, saffron	Spices, flavor enhancement, cooking
Herbals (medicinal)	Plant products used for prevention and/or treatment of disease, and for monitoring health; also called "phytomedicines"	Evening primrose oil, St. John's wort, Asian ginseng, chamomile, echinacea, gingko, green tea, valerian, yohimbe, and many others	Multiple uses as antioxidants, nutritional supplements, vitamins, minerals, trace elements, and many others
Nutraceuticals (Bioceuticals)	A food or fortified food product	Vitamins, minerals, milk, fortified dairy products, cereals, herbals, and many others	Nutritional supplementation and disease prevention
Supplements (dietary)	A manufactured product for adding to the diet; to correct deficiencies and maintain health, either from food sources or synthetic manufacture; in pill, capsule, tablet, or liquid form	Glucosamine (cartilage and bone health), vitamin D, calcium (bone health), probiotics, fish oils, and many others	Cartilage and bone health, collagen health, dietary deficiency states, muscle loss, bodybuilding, and others (Note: FDA rules prohibit claims for actually treating these conditions)

Concerning products of these four types of current interest to mental health practitioners and providers, specifically including products which have been shown to be effective through randomized controlled trials (RCTs, the "gold standard" for studies of safety and efficacy)—but rarely in terms of FDA approvals. Table 6.3 gives the clinical indication of some RCT-approved products, the category of the product, and examples of the product.

Table 6.3 Selected natural products proven effective through RCT testing

Clinical indication of the product	Category of the product	Examples of the product
Depression (off-label)	Vitamin (dietary supplement)	L-methyl folate (Deplin®), a "medical food" by prescription; folic acid preparations (OTC)
Depression, PMDD, smoking cessation (all off-label)	Essential amino acid (dietary supplement)	L-tryptophan; OTC preparations
Depression (unipolar, bipolar; off-label); hypertriglyceridemia (FDA-approved)	Fatty acid (dietary supplement)	Omega-3 fatty acids (fish oil); various OTC preparations; Lavazza® for hypertriglyceridemia
Depression, osteoarthritis cirrhosis, fatty liver disease (all off-label)	Essential amino acid (dietary supplement)	S-adenosyl-L-methionine (SAME); various OTC preparations
Depression, mild-to-moderate (off-label)	Botanical	St. John's wort; various OTC preparations
Depression for low vitamin D levels (off-label)	Nutraceutical (vitamin; dietary supplement)	Vitamin D; various OTC preparations
Insomnia and jetlag symptoms (off-label)	Pineal gland hormone (dietary supplement)	Pineal gland hormone, present in many foods; various OTC preparations
Trichotillomania, nail biting, skin picking, OCD (all off-label)	Semi-essential amino acid congener (dietary supplement)	N-acetylcysteine (NAC); various OTC preparations. Adjunctive to SSRIs in OCD and related conditions.

Adapted from Puzantian and Carlat (2020)

A "cook's tour" of the vast and parallel (to psychopharmacotherapy) world of natural products can only touch on salient features of that world; that has been the purpose of this chapter. "Take-away" messages for the reader of this *Primer* are:

- **Do not** underestimate the popularity, prevalence, and potential good that these varied products can do for patients/clients requiring mental health professional care and treatment,

  but

- **Do** be aware of the largely unregulated nature and scope of these varied products and the potential harm they can cause patients/clients from adverse and undesired ("side") effects,

  and

- In that vein, **do** be aware that by relying on natural products to the exclusion of psychopharmacotherapeutic agents, when indicated, some patients/clients may not receive the benefit they need from their natural products,

  and

- **Do** be aware, again, of the enormous popularity of these natural products and of CAM: Patients/clients are also aware of this popularity. They will often ask their treating mental health professionals about BHNSs, and make suggestions to those professionals about their using these products. In other words, be forewarned and be prepared!

A Note on References

Rather than burdening the reader with excessive and detailed references and citations in this *Primer*, given below are particularly useful selected references. In addition, other specific references and citations will be given in parentheses throughout the *Primer*. For further information and details about any topics presented and discussed in this book, the interested reader is referred not only to the following list of selected references but also to applicable textbooks, monographs, electronic databases, print articles and materials, internet sources, and other applicable resources.

Selected References

- Black DW, Andreasen NC. Introductory textbook of psychiatry. 6th ed. American Psychiatric Publishing, Inc.; 2014. (A solid basic textbook of psychiatry.)
- Multiple Authors. Diagnostic and statistical manual of mental health disorders (*DSM-5*). 5th ed. American Psychiatry Association, Inc.; 2013. (This book is the controversial "bible" for primarily American and Canadian psychiatric diagnoses.)
- The comparable international work to the *DSM-5* is currently the 2019 International Classification of Diseases (*ICD-10*). 10th ed. World Health Organization. (The *ICD-11* was due for adoption in 2020.)
- Frances A. Saving normal: an insider's revolt against out-of-control psychiatric diagnosis, big pharma, and the medicalization of ordinary life. Harper Collins Publishers: 2013. (The subtitle says it all! See Chap. 4 in this *Primer*.)
- Ghaemi SN. Clinical psychopharmacology: principles and practice. Oxford University Press: 2019. (A scholarly, detailed, and lengthy overview of psychopharmacology, also covering social practice and research/methodologic aspects of the field.)
- Hales RE, Yudofsky ST, Roberts LW, et al., editors. The American Psychiatric Publishing textbook of psychiatry. 6th ed. American Psychiatric Publishing, Inc.; 2014. (A standard, detailed encyclopedic textbook tome, for reference. A seventh edition is available, copyright 2019, with updated coverage in a number of areas.)
- Harrington A. Mind fixers: psychiatry's troubled search for the biology of mental illness. W.W. Norton and Company; 2019. (A historical and scholarly review of the topic, including some of the same topics as *Saving Normal* listed above.)
- Puzantian T, Carlat DJ. Medication fact book for psychiatric practice. 6th ed. Carlat Publishing, LLC; 2020. (A very useful "cookbook" for psychotropic prescribing, conveniently organized and presented for the practitioner.)
- Watters E. Crazy like us: the globalization of the American psyche. Free Press; 2010. (Psychiatric diagnostic issues similar to those in *Saving Normal*, with an international focus.)

- Weil A. Mind over meds: know when drugs are necessary, when alternatives are better—and when to let your body heal on its own. Little, Brown and Company; 2017. (A balanced and holistic approach to pharmacology and psychopharmacology by the popular "guru" of these fields.)

Selected Internet References

With the surfeit of internet resources, websites of all imaginable types and quality, and numerous related electronic sources of information and data, the reader, clinician, researcher, and member of the public—patient/client or not—may easily become confused about where to go and what to accept in learning psychopharmacology and psychopharmacotherapy. In this vein, a productive way to navigate the bewildering array of such sources consists of dividing them into several categories, viz.

1. Refereed ("peer-reviewed;" "juried") scientific, technical, and professional journals, newsletters, and the like, including e-journals, e-newsletters, and other open-source e-publications. Selected examples include:

   - *Journal of Clinical Psychopharmacology* (peer-reviewed independent professional journal)
   - *Experimental & Clinical Psychopharmacology* (peer-reviewed professional journal of the American Psychological Association)
   - *Journal of Psychopharmacology* (peer-reviewed professional journal of the British Association for Psychopharmacology)
   - *Psychopharmacology* (Berlin/Heidelberg; Springer Publications)

2. Government and academic/research institutions, publications and e-publications and associated websites. Selected examples include:

   - National Institute of Mental Health (NIMH) website, affiliated institutes, programs, centers, websites, and publications (electronic and print)
   - National Institute on Alcoholism and Alcohol Abuse (NIAAA) website, affiliated institutes, programs and centers, and websites and publications (electronic and print)
   - National Institute on Drug Abuse (NIDA) website, affiliated institutes, centers, programs and websites, and publications (electronic and print)
   - Canadian Centre on Substance Abuse (CCSA), affiliated programs and publications (electronic and print)
   - National Center on Addiction and Substance Abuse at Columbia University (NCASACU), programs and publications (electronic and print)

3. Journals, magazines, societies, and associated websites. Selected examples include:

- *Psychology Today*
- *Scientific American*
- *Scientific American Mind*

As a practical matter, in researching particular topics electronically in psychopharmacology/psychopharmacotherapy, the logical rule—as with everything else— is to search for topic(s), keyword(s), and the like on a search engine, then to narrow the search with entries given by the search engine. An important factor to keep in mind here is the reliability, accuracy, and quality of the source: Sources from (1) and (2)—above—are considered more reliable than those in (3), generally. Those in (3), in turn, are generally considered more reliable than personal blogs, newsletters, product websites, company websites, and the like.

Part II
Therapies That May Involve Psychopharmacology/ Psychopharmacotherapy

Chapter 7
A Selective Overview of Therapies in Mental Health Care

Current therapies or treatment approaches and modalities in mental health care may be broadly divided into two categories, viz., (1) "Psychotherapies" and (2) "Somatic Therapies." For present purposes, these modalities may be summarized as follows:

- **Psychotherapies** focus on verbal, psychological, and cognitive interactions and discussion, conscious and unconscious (i.e., of which the patient/client is and is not overtly aware, respectively), between the treating professional and the patient/client. Theoretically, these psychotherapeutic techniques bring about symptom relief and personal change through that interactive process, whether didactic (i.e., counseling, and giving advice), through insight on the patient's/client's part, or through behavioral techniques (i.e., using specific techniques based on learning theory to produce specific changes in undesired and dysfunctional behaviors, thereby alleviating problematic symptoms). This therapeutic approach relies heavily on the respective roles and expectations of the treated ("patient/client") and the treater ("therapist"): Those roles and expectations, in turn, are described in technical terms as "transference" on the part of the treated and "countertransference" on the part of the treater.
- **Somatic therapies**, on the other hand, follow the biomedical orientation of doing something to or putting something (e.g., psychotropic medications) into a client's/patient's body ("soma," from the Latin) in order to bring about a desired change in that individual's mood state, cognition, emotion or affect, mental state, and so forth, through manipulation of the patient's/client's physiology. Although a patient's/client's attitude and emotional condition do influence their response to the administration of such "somatic" interventions to some extent, the primary effect in the patient/client is intended to be the physiologic change brought about by the somatic intervention itself and not by the transference/countertransference effects and interactions of the patient/client and treating professional.

As a practical matter, a myriad of psychotherapies and somatic therapies exists, some frequently and infrequently practiced. A compendium of such treatments from

© The Author(s), under exclusive license to Springer Nature
Switzerland AG 2022
D. P. Greenfield, *Psychopharmacology for Nonpsychiatrists*,
https://doi.org/10.1007/978-3-030-82507-2_7

as long ago as 1980 identified over 250 different types of psychotherapies (Herink R. The psychotherapy handbook: the A to Z guide to more than 250 different therapies used today. New American Library; 1980) and a more recent text identified 12 such therapies in general use (Corsini RJ, Wedding D, editors. Current psychotherapies. 6th ed. Brooks Cole; 2000).

The purpose of this volume is not to provide a detailed or comprehensive review of all types of psychotherapies and somatic therapies. However, for present purposes, the reader should be aware of the place of psychopharmacology or—in treatment terminology—"pharmacotherapy/psychopharmacotherapy" in the universe of psychiatric and psychological treatments, given the focus of this book on one particular type of somatic treatment, namely "psychopharmacology." (See Tables 7.1 and 7.2).

Table 7.1 An overview of psychotherapies

Non-behavioral therapies
Adlerian psychotherapy
Asian psychotherapies
Couples therapy
Existential psychotherapy
Gestalt therapy
Insight-oriented/exploratory psychotherapy
Interpersonal therapy
Marital and family therapy
Multimodal therapy
Person-centered therapy
"Primal scream" therapy
Psychoanalysis
Self-help recovery group therapy such as alcoholics anonymous (AA) and narcotics anonymous (NA)
Supportive/relationship psychotherapy
Others
Behavioral therapies
Behavior modification
Cognitive behavioral therapy (CBT)
Dialectical behavioral therapy (DBT)
Hypnosis/hypnotherapy
Rational emotive behavior therapy
Mindfulness and meditation
Others

Table 7.2 An overview of somatic therapies

Psychopharmacotherapy
Brain stimulation therapies (electroshock therapies)
Electroconvulsive therapy (ECT)/electroshock therapy (EST)
Deep brain stimulation (DBS)
Transcranial magnetic stimulation (TMS)
Vagus nerve stimulation (VNS)
Magnetic seizure therapy (MST): experimental
Phototherapy/light therapy
For seasonal affective disorder syndrome (SADS): *DSM-5* specifier
Psychosurgery (brain surgery)
Coma therapies (historic)
Insulin coma therapy (ICT)/insulin shock therapy (IST): no longer used
Analeptic (seizure inducing) therapy/Metrazol therapy: no longer used

A Note on References

Rather than burdening the reader with excessive and detailed references and citations in this *Primer*, given below are particularly useful selected references. In addition, other specific references and citations will be given in parentheses throughout the *Primer*. For further information and details about any topics presented and discussed in this book, the interested reader is referred not only to the following list of selected references but also to applicable textbooks, monographs, electronic databases, print articles and materials, internet sources, and other applicable resources.

Selected References

- Black DW, Andreasen NC. Introductory textbook of psychiatry. 6th ed. American Psychiatric Publishing, Inc.; 2014. (A solid basic textbook of psychiatry.)
- Multiple Authors. Diagnostic and statistical manual of mental health disorders (*DSM-5*). 5th ed. American Psychiatry Association, Inc.; 2013. (This book is the controversial "bible" for primarily American and Canadian psychiatric diagnoses.)
- The comparable international work to the *DSM-5* is currently the 2019 International Classification of Diseases (*ICD-10*). 10th ed. World Health Organization. (The *ICD-11* was due for adoption in 2020.)
- Frances A. Saving normal: an insider's revolt against out-of-control psychiatric diagnosis, big pharma, and the medicalization of ordinary life. Harper Collins Publishers: 2013. (The subtitle says it all! See Chap. 4 in this *Primer*.)

- Ghaemi SN. Clinical psychopharmacology: principles and practice. Oxford University Press: 2019. (A scholarly, detailed, and lengthy overview of psychopharmacology, also covering social practice and research/methodologic aspects of the field.)
- Hales RE, Yudofsky ST, Roberts LW, et al., editors. The American Psychiatric Publishing textbook of psychiatry. 6th ed. American Psychiatric Publishing, Inc.; 2014. (A standard, detailed encyclopedic textbook tome, for reference. A seventh edition is available, copyright 2019, with updated coverage in a number of areas.)
- Harrington A. Mind fixers: psychiatry's troubled search for the biology of mental illness. W.W. Norton and Company; 2019. (A historical and scholarly review of the topic, including some of the same topics as *Saving Normal* listed above.)
- Puzantian T, Carlat DJ. Medication fact book for psychiatric practice. 6th ed. Carlat Publishing, LLC; 2020. (A very useful "cookbook" for psychotropic prescribing, conveniently organized and presented for the practitioner.)
- Watters E. Crazy like us: the globalization of the American psyche. Free Press; 2010. (Psychiatric diagnostic issues similar to those in *Saving Normal*, with an international focus.)
- Weil A. Mind over meds: know when drugs are necessary, when alternatives are better—and when to let your body heal on its own. Little, Brown and Company; 2017. (A balanced and holistic approach to pharmacology and psychopharmacology by the popular "guru" of these fields.)

Selected Internet References

With the surfeit of internet resources, websites of all imaginable types and quality, and numerous related electronic sources of information and data, the reader, clinician, researcher, and member of the public—patient/client or not—may easily become confused about where to go and what to accept in learning psychopharmacology and psychopharmacotherapy. In this vein, a productive way to navigate the bewildering array of such sources consists of dividing them into several categories, viz.

1. Refereed ("peer-reviewed;" "juried") scientific, technical, and professional journals, newsletters, and the like, including e-journals, e-newsletters, and other open-source e-publications. Selected examples include:

   - *Journal of Clinical Psychopharmacology* (peer-reviewed independent professional journal)
   - *Experimental & Clinical Psychopharmacology* (peer-reviewed professional journal of the American Psychological Association)
   - *Journal of Psychopharmacology* (peer-reviewed professional journal of the British Association for Psychopharmacology)
   - *Psychopharmacology* (Berlin/Heidelberg; Springer Publications)

2. Government and academic/research institutions, publications and e-publications and associated websites. Selected examples include:

- National Institute of Mental Health (NIMH) website, affiliated institutes, programs, centers, websites, and publications (electronic and print)
- National Institute on Alcoholism and Alcohol Abuse (NIAAA) website, affiliated institutes, programs and centers, and websites and publications (electronic and print)
- National Institute on Drug Abuse (NIDA) website, affiliated institutes, centers, programs and websites, and publications (electronic and print)
- Canadian Centre on Substance Abuse (CCSA), affiliated programs and publications (electronic and print)
- National Center on Addiction and Substance Abuse at Columbia University (NCASACU), programs and publications (electronic and print)

3. Journals, magazines, societies, and associated websites. Selected examples include:

- *Psychology Today*
- *Scientific American*
- *Scientific American Mind*

As a practical matter, in researching particular topics electronically in psychopharmacology/ psychopharmacotherapy the logical rule—as with everything else—is to search for topic(s), keyword(s), and the like on a search engine, then to narrow the search with entries given by the search engine. An important factor to keep in mind here is the reliability, accuracy, and quality of the source: Sources from (1) and (2)—above—are considered more reliable than those in (3), generally. Those in (3), in turn, are generally considered more reliable than personal blogs, newsletters, product websites, company websites, and the like.

Chapter 8
Psychotherapies and Counseling

In an insightful essay in *The New York Times* entitled "About That Mean Streak of Yours: Psychiatry Can Only Do So Much (When Nastiness Is A Personality Trait, Not A Sign of Mental Illness)," psychiatrist Richard A. Friedman offered the comment that "It's not fashionable in our therapy-friendly nation, where people who behave obnoxiously are assumed to have a treatable psychiatric problem until proven otherwise. Nothing in the human experience is beyond the power of psychiatry to diagnose or fix, it seems." He continues the essay by presenting several case examples of people—patients, actually—who should be considered "bad," not "mad," and concludes that "To put it another way, some medically ill patients can be mean or bad just like anyone else, and this is not a problem for psychiatry to fix" (Friedman R. "About That Mean Streak of Yours." *The New York Times*, February 6, 2007).

For those legions of other troubled people, many different types of what current parlance calls "mental health providers" are available to see to their needs, and many different ways for those "providers" to accomplish that goal. Historically, one of the earliest of those ways—after prehistoric neurosurgical techniques—was what has variously been called "therapy," "psychotherapy," "talk therapy," and "counseling." Those types of mental health treatments are the subject of this chapter.

As described in Chap. 7 ("An Overview of Therapies in Mental Health Care"), many different types of therapy are available to the disturbed public, far too many to be treated in detail in this chapter. Therefore, distinguishing broadly, between "nonbehavioral" and "behavioral" (see Table 7.1) and between "individual" and "group" psychotherapies, this chapter will present an overview of these therapies, focusing on those used most prevalently in current mental health practice.

© The Author(s), under exclusive license to Springer Nature
Switzerland AG 2022
D. P. Greenfield, *Psychopharmacology for Nonpsychiatrists*,
https://doi.org/10.1007/978-3-030-82507-2_8

In current mental health practice, shaped and directed by such practical factors as insurance reimbursement limitations, time limitations, non-availability in person (due to the coronavirus social distancing as of this writing) and financial restrictions, many of these therapies are combined with others (such as pharmacotherapy), in the interest of better and greater treatment outcomes and greater cost efficiency. These so-called "combination approaches" have been mentioned in Chap. 3 and 4 and will be revisited in Chap. 13.

Non-behavioral Psychotherapies

Table 8.1 depicts a continuum going from those non-behavioral individual therapies considered the least structured and didactic to those considered the most structured and didactic, with examples of psychotherapies of intermediate levels of structure in between. The following section elaborates on these individual non-behavioral psychotherapies.

Table 8.1 Continuum of non-behavioral individual psychotherapies (least structured to most structured)

Level of structure	Type of psychotherapy
Least structured	Psychoanalysis
	Psychodynamic (exploratory; insight-oriented) psychotherapy
	Supportive (rational) psychotherapy
	Brief short-term dynamic psychotherapy
	Interpersonal psychotherapy (IPT)
	Multimodal therapy
Most structured	Individual counseling

A limiting case on the unstructured end of the above continuum is classical Freudian "psychoanalysis." This treatment modality is derived from the discoveries and theories of the nineteenth century intuitively regarded by most individuals as the caricature of mental health treatment. While "rules" and "techniques" do exist in psychoanalytic practice, the role of the psychoanalyst or analyst is much less engaged in interactions with the patient than is the case with other psychotherapies. The psychoanalytic technique of "free association" (the patient/client speaks about whatever is on their mind in as uncensored and free-flowing way as possible, with minimal disturbance "on the couch" to the patient as possible) is the paradigmatic way in which psychoanalysis is conducted. Through the slow and painstaking insight gained independently by the patient/client, with periodic interpretation but little guidance by the psychoanalyst, progress and understanding come to the patient/client—often through frequent therapy sessions and a lengthy (years, not months) course of treatment—in dealing with such psychoanalytically labeled impediments as conflicts, resistances, and blocks. This is a slow, often difficult, expensive, and infrequently used treatment modality, historically important as a basis, or formulation for a number of schools and practices of psychotherapy (especially non-behavioral approaches) but not extensively used in current cost-conscious mental healthcare practices.

Variants of Freudian psychoanalysis are also practiced, such as Adlerian psychotherapy, Jungian analysis, Reichian analysis, and others. They all derive from the same era (late nineteenth and early twentieth century), and all represent "schools of thought" developed and promoted by their founders.

Somewhat more structured than psychoanalysis is "psychodynamic psychotherapy," also known as "exploratory psychotherapy" and "insight-oriented psychotherapy." Unlike the "schools" of psychoanalysis just described, psychodynamic psychotherapy is not associated with any particular founder or author, and as a practical matter, uses many of the same principles as psychoanalysis, albeit in an adulterated way. The use of such concepts as "transference" (the sum total of feelings and attitudes of patients toward the therapist in the context of the therapist–patient relationship, whether realistic or symbolic of psychological issues in the patient's life), "countertransference" (the converse of transference), "resistance" (unclear and/or unconscious reasons for a patient's lack of progress in treatment), the "therapeutic alliance" (a positive and productive treatment relationship between the patient and the therapist which, if not present, needs to be explored in therapy), and others derived from psychoanalytic principles characterizes "psychoanalytic psychotherapy." Like psychoanalysis, psychoanalytic psychotherapy tends to be of long term and not rigidly structured.

Next on the continuum of non-behavioral psychotherapies (Table 8.1) is "supportive (relational) psychotherapy." This approach is less intense and more structured than the two psychoanalytic approaches just discussed and involves more direct engagement by the therapist than do the psychoanalytic and psychodynamic approaches. The involvement of the therapist in the therapist–patient/client relationship includes giving the patient/client active encouragement, counseling, and advice, and—as the name indicates—active support and endorsement of the patient's/client's needs and plans, when appropriate. (This is a very different approach from that of the "technical neutrality" of the psychoanalyst, who serves as an interpreter of thoughts and ideas which originate with the patient and which are neither encouraged nor discouraged by the psychoanalyst. In that respect, another school of non-behavioral psychotherapy entitled "person-centered therapy," founded and promoted by the psychologist Carl Rogers, Ph.D., also focuses almost exclusively on the patient as the source of ideas and content for the therapy.)

Maintenance of appropriate boundaries and roles is important in this type of therapy, in that, for example, if the patient/client comes to rely excessively on the support and advice of the therapist, the patient's/client's autonomy could be undermined, and the positive effects of the therapy similarly diminished. An extreme example of what has been called "boundary erosion" could lead to inappropriate intimacy, and even sexual relations between the patient/client and the therapist, originating from either party, or consensually.

Brief dynamic psychotherapy, or short-term dynamic psychotherapy, is the next type of non-behavioral psychotherapy depicted in the continuum of Table 8.1. This type of therapy uses the principles of psychoanalysis and dynamic psychotherapy in a more concentrated and shorter time course than the other two approaches. Practically speaking, a specific number (usually fewer than 25) of treatment sessions is allotted, and specific treatment goals (such as overcoming a work inhibition) are articulated, with specific milestones identified to be accomplished during the course of treatment. The focus of treatment is on more circumscribed goals than in longer term treatment approaches. Intervention and feedback from the therapist are more frequent, direct, and didactic than in the longer term treatment approaches. Historically, an impetus for the development of this approach to treatment has been economic. As a practical matter, circumscribed and time-limited psychotherapeutic approaches have been shown to be cost-effective and efficient as measured and determined in a variety of ways, especially in many instances, when combined with psychopharmacotherapy (see Chap. 13 in this *Primer*).

Following brief dynamic psychotherapy on the continuum of Table 8.1 is interpersonal psychotherapy (IPT). IPT was developed in the 1990s as a practical and focused approach at first directed toward the treatment of non-psychotic depression. IPT addresses current psychological signs and symptoms of patient/client by linking such symptoms to one (or more) of several aspects of depression considered important to treatment (these are grief, role dispute, role transition, and interpersonal defects). In directed psychotherapy sessions on a short-term basis, applicable aspects of the patient's/client's depression are addressed, identified, and understood in a concrete and straightforward way in order to enable them to cope effectively with their troublesome symptomatology. In focusing on signs and symptoms in a "here and now" way; in not focusing on psychodynamic and historical potential "causes" of depressive symptomatology; and in using a structured and time-limited approach, IPT is similar to the focused approach which characterizes the behavioral psychotherapies, described below.

Multimodal therapy is a broad-based, systematic, and structured approach to psychotherapy which uses a wide variety of techniques and methods, to address both the multiple problems and problem areas of a given patient with **multiple modalities** (hence, the term multimodal). The acronym BASIC ID (which stands for Behavior, Affect, Sensation, Imagery, Cognitive, Interpersonal Relationships, and Drugs/Biology, including nutrition, hygiene, and exercise) conveys the broad range of assessment and intervention in multimodal therapy. As the next position in the continuum of Table 8.1, multimodal therapy is both highly structured and short-term. It is intended to address the many symptoms and problem areas found in many mental health patients, regardless of the patient's/client's specific underlying psychiatric diagnosis.

Finally, the most structured and didactic type of psychotherapy presented in Table 8.1 is called "individual counseling." Although that particular term may be used in a variety of ways in the various mental health professions, its use here is intended to convey the notion that "counseling" involves the didactic giving of advice ("counsel") from the informed and experienced mental health professional to the uninformed (or less informed) and inexperienced (or less experienced) patient/client. This process necessarily has less interactive give and take between counselor and patient than do other psychotherapies, even though a therapist–patient/client relationship exists, and such phenomena as role, role expectation, transference, and countertransference also exist in this type of non-behavioral psychotherapy.

In this discussion of non-behavioral therapies, so far, I have dealt only with **individual** psychotherapies. To complete this part of this chapter without going into unnecessary detail, I will conclude this section of this chapter with a discussion of therapies involving more than one individual at a time, specifically couples therapy, group therapy, and marriage and family therapy.

Starting with couples therapy, this modality and that of marriage and family therapy should be of considerable interest to the family or primary care-oriented practitioner. This is so because referrals of patients/clients for that type of treatment as well as evaluations by mental health professionals in those disciplines often constitute a significant focus of attention for those practitioners. Couples therapy—which may be defined as "…a format of intervention involving both members of a dyad, in which the focus of intervention is the problematic irrational patterns of the couple…" (Retvo et al. Couples and family therapy. In Hales RE, editor. The APP textbook of psychiatry. 5th ed. APP, Inc.; 2008)—is generally short-term, focused on dysfunctional aspects of the relationship between the couple (such as poor communication), and practical, in the sense of attempting to help the troubled couple deal with concrete problems. It is worth noting that with changing cultural mores, the term "couple" no longer necessarily refers to a paired relationship between a man and a woman of about the same age and of the same sociocultural and ethnic background. In this age of easing sociocultural and ethnic constraints, and incredibly rapid and broad electronic communication (instant messaging, texting, emailing, social networking, relationship websites, computer dating, and so forth), "coupling" can occur in an incredible variety of ways, with a potentially wide array of problems.

Conceptually, family therapy and couples therapy are similar endeavors, with individuals beyond the basic dyad—parents, children, and members of the dyad's extended family—included in therapy, to the extent that they contribute to family problems or to what is known in the field as "family pathology." Similar issues of poor communication, poor support, and connections among families and couples, dysfunctional problem-solving, sexual problems, different approaches to family and couples conflicts, and the like, are addressed in this type of psychotherapy.

Group therapy in concept is similar to couples therapy and marriage and family therapy, in that the focus is on more than one person. In the case of group therapy, the members of the therapeutic group go beyond intimates (couples therapy) and family members (marriage and family therapy) to include individuals who start out as strangers and whose initial common bond is membership in the group. Group settings in non-therapeutic settings—work, school, clubs, professional societies, and so forth—are ubiquitous, and although not always the case, membership in a cohesive and supportive group can be very invigorating and enhancing for its members. Therapeutic groups, or "support groups" in medical contexts, take advantage of this closeness and have been shown over the years to help their members succeed and do well in life, even in such non-psychological, medical, and somatic areas as increased breast cancer survival, increased malignant melanoma survival, and other types of cancer survival. A variety of therapeutic groups is found in inpatient, outpatient, partial hospital, and other treatment settings, involving patients (i.e., group members) with a wide array of psychiatric diagnoses and the full range of levels of impairment, or symptomatology (i.e., from fully functional—the "worried well"—to the overly and fully psychotic and dysfunctional). The core approaches to group psychotherapy in all of these types of groups involve support and positive regard for the group and its members, attitudes of acceptance toward group members, cohesiveness of the group, encouragement by members for other members to participate in the group process, and willingness of the members to change as a result of that learning, among many other such features.

In this vein, although I will not discuss the effectiveness of a wide range and variety of non-professionally led or supervised therapeutic groups—known as "self-help" groups, or "recovery" groups, such as Alcoholics Anonymous (AA), Gamblers Anonymous (GA), Narcotics Anonymous (NA), Sexaholics Anonymous (SA), Parents Without Partners, Compassionate Friends, Overeaters Anonymous (OA), and many others—I emphasize and endorse their widespread availability, low or non-existent cost, and widespread community acceptance, especially in the addictive orders (see Chap. 5 in this *Primer*). The group therapy principles of cohesiveness, a common goal, acceptance of the group, willingness to learn from the group, and many other such features also apply to these self-help groups.

I reiterate—a point made in Table 7.1 of Chap. 7 in this book—that schools and modalities of psychotherapeutic treatment, non-behavioral and behavioral alike, are numerous and that a detailed discussion of them is well beyond the scope and scale of this book. For further information and details, the interested reader is referred to applicable articles, electronic databases, internet references, textbooks, monographs, and the like in these areas.

Behavioral Psychotherapies

As is the case with non-behavioral psychotherapies, the behavioral therapies come in a wide variety and range of types. In this section, I will focus on a selected set of behavioral therapies, as listed in Table 8.2. As with the non-behavioral psychotherapies, a full discussion of behavioral psychotherapies is well beyond the nature and scope of this book. To research this topic further, the interested reader is also referred to applicable articles, electronic databases, internet references, textbooks, monographs, and the like in these areas.

Table 8.2 Behavioral therapies	Behavior (modification) therapy
	Rational emotive behavior therapy (REBT)
	Cognitive behavioral therapy (CBT)
	Dialectical behavioral therapy (DBT)
	Hypnosis/hypnotherapy
	Eye movement desensitization and reprocessing (EMDR)
	Mindfulness and meditation
	Metacognitive therapy
	Many others

Behavioral Therapy (Generally)

The common thread of behavioral therapies is the root of their treatment techniques in psychological learning theory, including the "classical conditioning" paradigm of the nineteenth century Russian physiologist, Ivan Pavlov and the twentieth-century "operant conditioning" paradigm of the American psychologist, Burroughs F. (B.F.) Skinner, and other approaches containing features of both. In these paradigms, the effect of stimulating the organism (the patient/client or person, or "black box," for present purposes) is paramount, without the need for a detailed (or psychodynamic, for present purposes) understanding of what happens in the "black box." The "organism" somehow processes stimuli, receiving them and turning them into predictable, measurable, and productive responses and behaviors. The behavior is "modified" without the strong need to "understand" it on a psychological or neurobiological level.

According to both classical and operant conditioning paradigms, specific changes in the initial stimulation subsequent "reinforcers" (reinforcing stimuli), whether introduced from outside the organism or from within the organism, can shape subsequent behaviors in the organism in desirable ways, if properly done.

An example of classical, or Pavlovian, conditioning is the temporal pairing of an unconditioned stimulus (meat powder, which will cause a dog to salivate reflexively, without any previous training) with a conditioning stimulus (the ring of a bell, which will not cause a dog to salivate, but is the stimulus which is to become an unconditioned stimulus in this experimental model): Given the right timing and intensity (of the two stimuli) factors, the conditioning stimulus will link with the unconditioned stimulus, cause the dog to salivate, become interchangeable with the unconditional stimulus, and eventually replace the unconditioned stimulus altogether.

An example of operant, or Skinnerian conditioning of clinical mental health significance, is the organism's substitution through therapy and training of positively reinforcing internal stimuli for negative such stimuli, with resulting positive effect, clinical improvement, and reduction of negative psychological signs and symptoms. In a clinical application, Dr. Martin Seligman's concept of "learned helplessness" which "…postulates that past experiences of real helplessness imbue the individual with the connection that future unpleasant situations will also be uncontrollable, and therefore, such situations are responded to by passivity, resignation, and depressive acceptance…" (Corsini RJ, Wedding D, editors. Current psychotherapies. 6th ed. Brooks Cole; 2000) is a good example of both classical and operant behavioral models. The substitution of positive—not helpless—percepts for these "…past experiences of real helplessness…" in a conscious, aware, and behavioral way enables the patient/client or person, to "unlearn" these negative percepts, and in conditioning parlance, to lessen the strength between the associations connecting the stimuli with responses. The depression, anxiety, fear (or other such impairing symptomatology) is lessened or even eliminated, and the patient/client feels better. In an applied clinical setting, treatment approaches using this model are broadly called behavioral therapy. Three specific historical schools of thoughts in these approaches (now subsumed under the broader school of "cognitive behavior therapy," or CBT, as discussed next) were called "applied behavior analysis," "neo-behaviorist meditational stimulus-response model," and "social-cognitive theory."

Rational-Emotive Behavior Therapy (REBT)

Historically, an important school of personality theory and behavioral psychotherapy is called rational-emotive behavior therapy, or REBT, developed by clinical psychologist, Albert Ellis, Ph.D., in the 1950s. Now subsumed by more current approaches in behavioral psychotherapies (especially CBT), the contribution brought to behavioral psychotherapy by REBT uses the assertion that (1) an individual's underlying **belief system**—rational or not—is an important determinant to their behavioral reaction, or response to a stimulus, on the one hand, and conversely that (2) this belief system is an important determinant to how that individual permits themselves to handle therapy. In Ellis' words:

> …when a highly charged emotion consequence follows a significant activity event (A), event A may seem to, but actually does not, cause C. Instead, emotional consequences are largely created by B—the individual's belief system. When an undesirable emotional consequence occurs, such as severe anxiety, this usually involves the person's irrational beliefs, and when these beliefs are effectively disputed (at point D), by challenging them rationally and behaviorally, the disturbed consequences are reduced. (Ellis A. Rational emotive therapy. In Corsini RJ, Wedding D, editors. Current psychotherapies. 6th ed. Brooks Cole; 2000)

Practically speaking, REBT is an eclectic type of behavioral therapy, using counseling, role-playing, desensitization, support, suggestion, assertiveness training, and other such techniques in a therapy described as similar to cognitive behavior therapy.

Cognitive Behavior Therapy

Currently, cognitive behavior therapy (CBT) is probably the most widely practiced form of all behavioral psychotherapies. CBT derives from the work of psychiatrist Aaron Beck, M.D. and his colleagues at the University of Pennsylvania, beginning in the 1960s. As described by Beck and his colleagues, this "…cognitive model for psychotherapy is grounded on the theory that there are characteristic errors in information processing in psychiatric disorders, and that these alterations in thought processes are closely linked to emotional reactions and dysfunctional behavior patterns…" (Wright JH, et al. Cognitive therapy. In Hales RE, et al., editors. The American Psychiatric Publishing textbook of psychiatry. APP, Inc.; 2008). Originally formulated as treatment for depression, CBT has been extended over the years to treat anxiety and panic disorders, phobias, psychoses, personality disorders, substance abuse disorders, eating disorders, bipolar disorders, and psychiatric symptomatology (such as anxiety and depression) secondary to a wide variety of medical conditions. A course of CBT starts with an interactive and problem-solving collaboration between the patient and the therapist, in which negative percepts, stimulus blocks to the patient's well-being and self-image, interpersonal conflicts, and other such problems and problem areas are identified (such "automatic thoughts" like "I always freeze in a new social situation," or "I can never please my partner"); made explicit (through concrete and explicit assignments, such as keeping a log or completing a workbook); and systematically altered through various (cognitive) exercises, active intervention and assistance by the therapist, and what has been called "collaborative empiricism" in the therapist–patient relationship. CBT is usually a short-term type of treatment, with concrete and specific goals identified, and behavioral treatment approaches applied, and with follow-up and "booster" courses of treatment as necessary, especially for patients with longstanding chronic conditions. As with a number of other types of therapy, CBT is "manual-based," with protocols, algorithms, instructions, and other such structured devices included in print and electronic instruction manuals for this therapy.

As a paradigm of behavioral approaches focusing on the "black box" of the patient and on practical goals and results of treatment, CBT has become popular and prevalent in a variety of mental health professions; has been extensively researched over the years and shown to be effective for many patients/clients; and is widely taught and practiced in many different mental health settings, both explicitly and as a treatment model for eclectic approaches to mental health treatment, often in combination with psychopharmacotherapy (see Chap. 13).

A variant of CBT which addresses a major public health problem—insomnia (see Chap. 4: "Anti-insomnia Agents")—is called cognitive behavior therapy for insomnia, or CBT-I. Using the principles of CBT (e.g., cognitive restructuring and psychoeducation) to start, this approach is considered a multicomponent type of treatment, in that in addition to CBT, it uses such additional sleep-inducing and sleep-maintaining techniques as stimulus (light, noise, ambient room temperature) control; sleep hygiene; sleep restricting and structuring (e.g., fixed bedtimes and wake-up times); relaxation training (e.g., breathing exercises); progressive muscle relaxation; autogenic training; biofeedback; hypnosis (see below, this chapter), meditation (see below, this chapter), and homework (e.g., using a sleep diary, for feedback).

For present purposes and for the reader of this book, CTB-I is generally a short-term (6-8 treatment sessions) and effective treatment modality not requiring "Anti-insomnia Agents" (Chap. 4) for primary insomnia (i.e., not a symptom of an underlying psychotic disorder such as anxiety or PTSD, sometimes requiring its own psychopharmacotherapy), which often can be administered by primary care professionals, without the need for referral to sleep medicine specialists.

Dialectical Behavior Therapy

Also classified as a brief psychotherapy, dialectical behavior therapy, or DBT, was developed by psychologist Marsha Linehan, Ph.D. in the early 1990s as a short-term, focused, and intense way to treat seriously troubled and difficult patients/clients (among others). Such patients/clients may include those with borderline personality disorder (see Chap. 2), suicidal patients/clients, patients/clients with addictions, impulsive patients/clients, and others. This approach uses short-term (brief), sequential interventions in an accepting therapeutic environment, in which the therapist, as a practical matter, endorses positive and productive behaviors, attitudes and beliefs, but discourages negative ones in a didactic and instructive way, as well as in an interactive ("dialectical") way. In the second edition of *What Works for Whom?* (Roth A, Fonagy P. Guilford Press; 2006) the authors report that DBT is more effective in modifying dysfunctional behaviors than in changing more global aspects of functioning, such as interpersonal relationships. This finding is expect-able in a behaviorally-oriented, goal-directed, and short-term-focused behavioral therapy geared toward modifying, or changing, specific identified behaviors.

Hypnosis and Hypnotherapy

Hypnosis and hypnotherapy probably have the most colorful and intriguing history of any school or type of psychotherapy, embodying both pre-scientific study and applications (such as "animal magnetism," Mesmerism, and parlor tricks—which still find spellbound crowds of observers at parties and other such events) and scientific applications. The mid-nineteenth century interest in states of split consciousness led to the systematic study of sleep and somnambulism (Zilboorg G, Henry G. A history of medical psychology. W.W. Norton and Company; 1941) by such iconic clinicians as Jean-Martin Charcot, Pierre Janet, Hippolyte Bernheim, and Sigmund Freud. These individuals used hypnosis as a means of studying these conditions, which later evolved to one of the two broad present-day applications of hypnosis, viz., diagnostic interviewing.

Currently, the two major areas of use of hypnosis/hypnotherapy in mental health are in diagnosis and therapy. In the latter applications, hypnosis/hypnotherapy may be considered the most structured and directed of the behavioral therapies in the list of Behavioral Psychotherapies in Table 8.2 (above). However, from the legal perspective (see Part III of this book), as a subset of the former diagnostic application of hypnosis—specifically in the forensic application of the hypnotic interview in detecting truth—the interest of the legal profession requires some knowledge of this intriguing subject.

Going back to 1896—the year of the first admission of hypnotic testimony as evidence in a court proceeding (Gravitz MA. First Admission (1846) of Hypnotic Testimony in Court. In American Journal of Clinical Hypnosis. American Society of Clinical Hypnosis; 2002)—hypnosis in the court room has fascinated onlookers, even though, generally, courts have been uniformly unwilling to admit the testimony of a person hypnotized while testifying. Requirements vary among venues about the circumstances and conditions under which information obtained under hypnosis may be admitted as evidence and how that information may be used in court proceedings: It behooves the legal practitioner to be familiar with these requirements in the venue in which such information might be used. However, from the clinical perspective, recent guidelines (Maldonado J, Spiegel D. Dissociative disorders. In Hales RE, et al., editors. The American Psychiatric Publishing textbook of psychiatry. APP, Inc.; 2008) suggest that a series of 17 detailed steps be followed by clinicians doing forensic hypnotic evaluations to be certain that proper clinical, ethical, and legal practices are observed. These requirements include obtaining the evaluee's informed consent, maintaining neutrality (not advocacy) during the evaluation, measuring the prospective subject's hypnotizability objectively, video recording all hypnotically-involved interactions, clarifying with evaluees the nature and scope of their expectations from hypnosis and others.

Advocacy and other such forensic/legal topics of interest to the mental health professional and the legal professional are discussed in Part III.

Eye Movement Desensitization and Reprocessing (EMDR)

Eye Movement Desensitization and Reprocessing (EMDR) is a behaviorally-oriented type of psychotherapy first developed by Francine Shapiro, Ph.D., a psychologist, in 1987, especially intended for and endorsed for the treatment of symptoms of post-traumatic stress disorder (PTSD: see Chaps. 1 and 2, and the *DSM-5*), along with other such exposure-based modalities as exposure therapy, trauma-focused cognitive behavior therapy, and others. The traumatic symptomatology to be treated by PTSD include anxiety (in this context, in earlier iterations of the *DSM*, PTSD was categorized as a subtype of anxiety disorder, not as a category of its own: "Trauma and stressor-related disorders;" see Chap. 1), depression, hypervigilance, avoidance (of the traumatic stressor environment), recurring nightmares of the traumatic event, flashbacks of the traumatic event, psychic numbing, feelings of detachment from others, generalized lack of interest, hypervigilance, dyssomnia, difficulty concentrating, irritability, guilt or shame, and others.

The technique of EMDR involves multiple structured treatment sessions with a trained EMDR therapist in which the patient/client focuses on the traumatic stimulus memory while simultaneously being exposed to a mental stimulus (eye movements, with EMDR) while through an unknown mechanism is associated with a dulling of the emotional impact and symptomatology of the memory of the traumatic stimulus. This treatment modality and its apparently adaptive "reprocessing" of negative and emotionally destructive traumatic memories is widely used in work with trauma victims, along with other similar modalities, including psychopharmacotherapy (currently, SSRIs and minipres [Prazosin®]: Sertraline [Zoloft®] and paroxetine [Paxil®] are FDA-approved for use with PTSD, and other SSRIs are also used, all to treat the target depression-related symptoms of PTSD; minipres [Prazosin®], an antihypertensive, is used off-label for nightmares in PTSD; see Chap. 4, "Anti-trauma Agents"), and combination therapies.

Mindfulness and Meditation

No discussion of psychotherapies would be complete without mindfulness and meditation. These techniques, known and practiced for hundreds of years if not longer, have become extremely popular in about the past 30 to 40 years, along with public enthusiasm about self-help, holistic health care, "patients/clients as consumers," patient/client autonomy, and other such trends (see Chap. 6). "Mindfulness," defined by one of its main spokespersons and proponents, Jon Kabat-Zinn, Ph.D., as "…paying attention in a particular way: on purpose, in the present moment and nonjudgmentally…" (Williams ME. Why every mind needs mindfulness. In TIME Special Edition: Mindfulness, The New Science of Health and Happiness. Time, Inc.; April 2017) describes a state of mind, attitude, and approach to life's problems. "Meditation" is a technique—or more correctly, a number of techniques—which helps the meditator to achieve a state of mindfulness. An important work in the "history" of Western meditation is Dr. Herbert Benson's (1974) *The Relaxation Response, First Edition*: As an academic cardiologist adept in applying meditation techniques to his practice, the popularity of Dr. Benson's book lent credibility to meditation and mindfulness in medical circles and established the effectiveness of these techniques in medical care for a wide range of conditions.

From the patient's/client's perspective, these techniques are without adverse ("side") effects, inexpensive, readily available, and even enjoyable. A full review of the types and techniques of mindfulness and meditations is beyond the scope of this brief review, and the interested reader is referred to myriad textbooks, articles, electronic databases, internet sources, and the like for further information and details about these prevalent, useful, and healthy practice.

Metacognitive Therapy

In the early 1990s, a type of behavioral therapy called "metacognitive therapy" (from the Greek: "meta," or "beyond;" and the Latin: "cognoscere," or "to think") was developed, focusing on how individuals **think** in contrast to what they **feel**. In that sense, this approach to psychological treatment was analogous to Seligman's "learned helplessness model of depression," in which the pattern or mechanism of depressed individual's thinking (i.e., "how they got there") took precedence over the depression symptomatology itself and lent itself to behavior intervention.

Similarly, the process of "catastrophizing" (i.e., "making a mountain out of a molehill," or "anticipating the worst") also applies to metacognitive therapy as the way for an affected individual to develop secondary concerns and defenses. In the case of anxiety, for example, such an individual may be worried that their worry will spin out of control and that they will "worry about worrying" to the point of psychological paralysis.

Enter metacognitive therapy: By offering patients/clients structured, task-oriented, practical, and concrete (i.e., behavioral) activities, such individuals are, in effect, distracted from their symptomatology (e.g., anxiety or depression) and diverted to focus on the activity, or task of their metacognitive therapy. Then, in theory, over time, the goal-directed and practical thinking (and its assorted lack of serious symptomatology) prevails, and takes over the affected individual's psyche, going forward.

While the above gives a very brief summary of metacognitive therapy, it is no substitute for a careful review of the literature, print sources, internet resources, consultation with practitioners, and the like, for the interested reader.

Psychotherapy and Counseling During the COVID Pandemic

The New York Times Sunday Review on October 25, 2020—during the early onset of the second wave of the pandemic in the United States—carried the following excerpt from an editorial by columnist Nicholas Kristof covering the mental health impact of the SARS-CoV-2 (or COVID-19) pandemic:

> ...More than 40% of adults reported in June [2020] that they were struggling with mental health, and 13% have begun or increased substance abuse, a CDC study found. More than one-quarter of young adults said they have seriously contemplated suicide.... (Kristof N. America and the Virus: 'A Colossal Failure of Leadership.' In *The New York Times*. 2020, October 22. https://www.nytimes.com/2020/10/22/opinion/sunday/coronavirus-united-states.html).

Without taking a deeper dive into the epidemiologic and clinical aspects of what is likely the most overwhelming biopsychosocial event in all our lifetimes, these data underscore that healthcare providers of all types are being and will continue to be called upon to minister to the needs of many of those currently impacted by the pandemic. This necessity will likely continue for many months to come, virtually (i.e., via telemedicine and teletherapy) and/or live, and with psychopharmacotherapy and/or counseling/psychotherapy.

Concerning pandemic-related psychotherapy and counseling, Osna Haller, Ph.D., a clinical psychologist and psychoanalyst (see section "Non-behavioral Psychotherapies") articulated three approaches to this public health issue in a recent guest lecture on October 22, 2020 given to physician assistant students attending the author's psychiatry course at Seton Hall University:

- Recognize and accept the varied and far-reaching effects of the COVID pandemic on the mental health of the entire population of the world.
- In psychotherapy and counseling, recognize and accept the resiliency of people in coping with stressors of the pandemic and incorporate that resiliency into treatment.
- As in any clinical situation, evaluate the patient's/client's therapeutic needs and conduct treatment accordingly, with (for example) modalities described in this chapter, and/or with clinically indicated psychopharmacotherapy. (Haller, O. Psychotherapy and Counseling during the COVID Pandemic. *Unpublished lecture*. October 22, 2020).

In a phrase often seen and heard since the pandemic began, "We're all in this together." The mental and physical damage which the pandemic has and will continue to wreak on all of us will continue to require the creative and hard work of healthcare professionals of all types for many individuals for a long time into the future.

A Note on References

Rather than burdening the reader with excessive and detailed references and citations in this *Primer*, given below are particularly useful selected references. In addition, other specific references and citations will be given in parentheses throughout the *Primer*. For further information and details about any topics presented and discussed in this book, the interested reader is referred not only to the following list of selected references but also to applicable textbooks, monographs, electronic databases, print articles and materials, internet sources, and other applicable resources.

Selected References

- Black DW, Andreasen NC. Introductory textbook of psychiatry. 6th ed. American Psychiatric Publishing, Inc.; 2014. (A solid basic textbook of psychiatry.)
- Multiple Authors. Diagnostic and statistical manual of mental health disorders (*DSM-5*). 5th ed. American Psychiatry Association, Inc.; 2013. (This book is the

controversial "bible" for primarily American and Canadian psychiatric diagnoses.)

- The comparable international work to the *DSM-5* is currently the 2019 International Classification of Diseases (*ICD-10*). 10th ed. World Health Organization. (The *ICD-11* was due for adoption in 2020.)
- Frances A. Saving normal: an insider's revolt against out-of-control psychiatric diagnosis, big pharma, and the medicalization of ordinary life. Harper Collins Publishers: 2013. (The subtitle says it all! See Chap. 4 in this *Primer*.)
- Ghaemi SN. Clinical psychopharmacology: principles and practice. Oxford University Press: 2019. (A scholarly, detailed, and lengthy overview of psychopharmacology, also covering social practice and research/methodologic aspects of the field.)
- Hales RE, Yudofsky ST, Roberts LW, et al., editors. The American Psychiatric Publishing textbook of psychiatry. 6th ed. American Psychiatric Publishing, Inc.; 2014. (A standard, detailed encyclopedic textbook tome, for reference. A seventh edition is available, copyright 2019, with updated coverage in a number of areas.)
- Harrington A. Mind fixers: psychiatry's troubled search for the biology of mental illness. W.W. Norton and Company; 2019. (A historical and scholarly review of the topic, including some of the same topics as *Saving Normal* listed above.)
- Puzantian T, Carlat DJ. Medication fact book for psychiatric practice. 6th ed. Carlat Publishing, LLC; 2020. (A very useful "cookbook" for psychotropic prescribing, conveniently organized and presented for the practitioner.)
- Watters E. Crazy like us: the globalization of the American psyche. Free Press; 2010. (Psychiatric diagnostic issues similar to those in *Saving Normal*, with an international focus.)
- Weil A. Mind over meds: know when drugs are necessary, when alternatives are better—and when to let your body heal on its own. Little, Brown and Company; 2017. (A balanced and holistic approach to pharmacology and psychopharmacology by the popular "guru" of these fields.)

Selected Internet References

With the surfeit of internet resources, websites of all imaginable types and quality, and numerous related electronic sources of information and data, the reader, clinician, researcher, and member of the public—patient/client or not—may easily become confused about where to go and what to accept in learning psychopharmacology and psychopharmacotherapy. In this vein, a productive way to navigate the bewildering array of such sources consists of dividing them into several categories, viz.

1. Refereed ("peer-reviewed;" "juried") scientific, technical, and professional journals, newsletters, and the like, including e-journals, e-newsletters, and other open-source e-publications. Selected examples include:

- *Journal of Clinical Psychopharmacology* (peer-reviewed independent professional journal)
- *Experimental & Clinical Psychopharmacology* (peer-reviewed professional journal of the American Psychological Association)
- *Journal of Psychopharmacology* (peer-reviewed professional journal of the British Association for Psychopharmacology)
- *Psychopharmacology* (Berlin/Heidelberg; Springer Publications)

2. Government and academic/research institutions, publications and e-publications and associated websites. Selected examples include:

- National Institute of Mental Health (NIMH) website, affiliated institutes, programs, centers, websites, and publications (electronic and print)
- National Institute on Alcoholism and Alcohol Abuse (NIAAA) website, affiliated institutes, programs and centers, and websites and publications (electronic and print)
- National Institute on Drug Abuse (NIDA) website, affiliated institutes, centers, programs and websites, and publications (electronic and print)
- Canadian Centre on Substance Abuse (CCSA), affiliated programs and publications (electronic and print)
- National Center on Addiction and Substance Abuse at Columbia University (NCASACU), programs and publications (electronic and print)

3. Journals, magazines, societies, and associated websites. Selected examples include:

- *Psychology Today*
- *Scientific American*
- *Scientific American Mind*

As a practical matter, in researching particular topics electronically in psychopharmacology/psychopharmacotherapy, the logical rule—as with everything else—is to search for topic(s), keyword(s), and the like on a search engine, then to narrow the search with entries given by the search engine. An important factor to keep in mind here is the reliability, accuracy, and quality of the source: Sources from (1) and (2)—above—are considered more reliable than those in (3), generally. Those in (3), in turn, are generally considered more reliable than personal blogs, newsletters, product websites, company websites, and the like.

Chapter 9
Somatic Therapies (Somatotherapies)

As described in the introductory chapter (Chap. 7, "An Overview of Therapies in Mental Health Care") to this part of this *Primer*, the common thread of somatic therapies is the notion of doing something (necessarily non-pharmacologic) to a patient's/client's body ("soma"), usually the brain, to bring about a lessening or amelioration of undesirable symptomatology (for present purposes, to "anti" undesired signs and symptoms), through manipulation of the patient's/client's physiology. In that sense, psychopharmacology/psychopharmacotherapy is considered one type of somatic therapy. Current terms used to describe these therapies include neuromodulation, brain stimulation techniques and recently electroceutical therapies, and neuropharmacologic somatic treatments.

Going back many years, other types of somatic therapies have been used. These include outmoded and outdated approaches (such as analeptic/seizure-inducing, or Metrazol® therapy; insulin shock therapy; dental and general surgical extraction; hemodialysis; and others).

Current such somatotherapies include the longstanding effective modality of seizure induction through electrical stimulation of the brain (electroconvulsive/electroshock therapy or ECT/EST); more recent variants of electrical and magnetic stimulation techniques (transcranial magnetic stimulation, or TMS, and repetitive TMS, or rTMS; vagal nerve stimulation, or VNS; and deep brain stimulation, or DBS); and even more recent experimental variants of these approaches (for examples: magnetic seizure therapy, or MST; transcutaneous electrical nerve stimulation (TENS), light therapy (phototherapy); and focal electrically administered seizure therapy, or FEAST). Table 9.1 summarizes these different therapies and their clinical indications.

D. P. Greenfield, *Psychopharmacology for Nonpsychiatrists*, https://doi.org/10.1007/978-3-030-82507-2_9

Table 9.1 Summary of somatic therapies (other than psychopharmacotherapy)

Therapy	Clinical indication(s)
Electroconvulsive/electroshock therapy (ECT/EST)	Depression, mania, catatonia
Transcranial magnetic stimulation (TMS); repetitive transcranial magnetic stimulation (rTMS)	Depression
Vagus nerve stimulation (VNS)	Treatment-resistant depression
Deep brain stimulation (DBS)	Treatment-resistant depression, Parkinson's disease, PTSD
Magnetic seizure therapy (MST)	Depression (experimental)
Focal electrically administered seizure therapy (FEAST)	Depression (experimental)
Transcranial direct current stimulation (tDCS)	Depression; substance abuse (experimental)
Transcutaneous electrical nerve stimulation (TENS)	Peripheral nerve pain relief

Adapted from Hales et al. (2014)

Without reiterating details of clinical indications, methodology and techniques, treatment outcome measures, and the like for these various somatic therapy modalities, several common features apply to all of them:

1. They recognize that the brain (and the central nervous system or CNS) is an electro-chemical body organ, that electrical impulse conduction is the core basis and function of the CNS, and that it operates by influencing this conduction.
2. The concomitant growth and development of neuroimaging techniques (e.g., neurosurgical placement of DBS electrodes) have contributed to a better scientific understanding of the mechanism of action of the therapies.
3. These therapies are usually used in conjunction with other therapies (e.g., psychopharmacotherapy in treating treatment-resistant depression) as supplementary treatments and not alone, sometimes providing synergistic interactive effects and dramatic patient/client clinical improvement.

Since this present *Primer* is not intended to be a comprehensive or detailed compendium of its subject matter, the reader is referred to works given in the Selected References for this chapter, as well as applicable monographs, books, articles, electronic databases, and current internet sources, for further information and details about somatic therapies.

A Note on References

Rather than burdening the reader with excessive and detailed references and citations in this *Primer*, given below are particularly useful selected references. In addition, other specific references and citations will be given in parentheses throughout the *Primer*. For further information and details about any topics presented and discussed in this book, the interested reader is referred not only to the following list of selected references but also to applicable textbooks, monographs, electronic databases, print articles and materials, internet sources, and other applicable resources.

Selected References

- Black DW, Andreasen NC. Introductory textbook of psychiatry. 6th ed. American Psychiatric Publishing, Inc.; 2014. (A solid basic textbook of psychiatry.)
- Multiple Authors. Diagnostic and statistical manual of mental health disorders (*DSM-5*). 5th ed. American Psychiatry Association, Inc.; 2013. (This book is the controversial "bible" for primarily American and Canadian psychiatric diagnoses.)
- The comparable international work to the *DSM-5* is currently the 2019 International Classification of Diseases (*ICD-10*). 10th ed. World Health Organization. (The *ICD-11* was due for adoption in 2020.)
- Frances A. Saving normal: an insider's revolt against out-of-control psychiatric diagnosis, big pharma, and the medicalization of ordinary life. Harper Collins Publishers: 2013. (The subtitle says it all! See Chap. 4 in this *Primer*.)
- Ghaemi SN. Clinical psychopharmacology: principles and practice. Oxford University Press: 2019. (A scholarly, detailed, and lengthy overview of psychopharmacology, also covering social practice and research/methodologic aspects of the field.)
- Hales RE, Yudofsky ST, Roberts LW, et al., editors. The American Psychiatric Publishing textbook of psychiatry. 6th ed. American Psychiatric Publishing, Inc.; 2014. (A standard, detailed encyclopedic textbook tome, for reference. A seventh edition is available, copyright 2019, with updated coverage in a number of areas.)
- Harrington A. Mind fixers: psychiatry's troubled search for the biology of mental illness. W.W. Norton and Company; 2019. (A historical and scholarly review of the topic, including some of the same topics as *Saving Normal* listed above.)
- Puzantian T, Carlat DJ. Medication fact book for psychiatric practice. 6th ed. Carlat Publishing, LLC; 2020. (A very useful "cookbook" for psychotropic prescribing, conveniently organized and presented for the practitioner.)
- Watters E. Crazy like us: the globalization of the American psyche. Free Press; 2010. (Psychiatric diagnostic issues similar to those in *Saving Normal*, with an international focus.)
- Weil A. Mind over meds: know when drugs are necessary, when alternatives are better—and when to let your body heal on its own. Little, Brown and Company; 2017. (A balanced and holistic approach to pharmacology and psychopharmacology by the popular "guru" of these fields.)

Selected Internet References

With the surfeit of internet resources, websites of all imaginable types and quality, and numerous related electronic sources of information and data, the reader, clinician, researcher, and member of the public—patient/client or not—may easily become confused about where to go and what to accept in learning psychopharmacology and psychopharmacotherapy. In this vein, a productive way to navigate the bewildering array of such sources consists of dividing them into several categories, viz.

1. Refereed ("peer-reviewed;" "juried") scientific, technical, and professional journals, newsletters, and the like, including e-journals, e-newsletters, and other open-source e-publications. Selected examples include:

   - *Journal of Clinical Psychopharmacology* (peer-reviewed independent professional journal)
   - *Experimental & Clinical Psychopharmacology* (peer-reviewed professional journal of the American Psychological Association)
   - *Journal of Psychopharmacology* (peer-reviewed professional journal of the British Association for Psychopharmacology)
   - *Psychopharmacology* (Berlin/Heidelberg; Springer Publications)

2. Government and academic/research institutions, publications and e-publications and associated websites. Selected examples include:

   - National Institute of Mental Health (NIMH) website, affiliated institutes, programs, centers, websites, and publications (electronic and print)
   - National Institute on Alcoholism and Alcohol Abuse (NIAAA) website, affiliated institutes, programs and centers, and websites and publications (electronic and print)
   - National Institute on Drug Abuse (NIDA) website, affiliated institutes, centers, programs and websites, and publications (electronic and print)
   - Canadian Centre on Substance Abuse (CCSA), affiliated programs and publications (electronic and print)
   - National Center on Addiction and Substance Abuse at Columbia University (NCASACU), programs and publications (electronic and print)

3. Journals, magazines, societies, and associated websites. Selected examples include:

   - *Psychology Today*
   - *Scientific American*
   - *Scientific American Mind*

As a practical matter, in researching particular topics electronically in psycho-pharmacology/psychopharmacotherapy, the logical rule—as with everything else—is to search for topic(s), keyword(s), and the like on a search engine, then to narrow the search with entries given by the search engine. An important factor to keep in mind here is the reliability, accuracy, and quality of the source: Sources from (1) and (2)—above—are considered more reliable than those in (3), generally. Those in (3), in turn, are generally considered more reliable than personal blogs, newsletters, product websites, company websites, and the like.

Part III
Forensic and Legal Applications of Psychopharmacology/ Psychopharmacotherapy

Chapter 10
Overview

For practicing attorneys, law professors, paralegals, and other legal professionals—regardless of their work and specialties—properties and effects of "licit" (legitimately prescribed by medical providers) and "street" (illicit substances or prescribed medications diverted from their intended use) psychotropic agents may be relevant to clients with psychiatric backgrounds and histories, to an understanding of clients' mental states at different periods of time, and to clients' ability to work with counsel in a variety of ways. Table 10.1 presents a broad overview of these potential applications of psychopharmacology to the law.

To be more specific and to flesh out the extent to which psychopharmacology figures in the law, a computer-based LexisNexis® Academic search, restricted to 10 years (1999–2009), of approximately 31,000 reported appellate cases in federal and state jurisdictions[1] of those cases, revealed a large number—about 6200, or approximately 20% of the 31,000—in which psychopharmacologic drugs and medications (as discussed in this *Primer*) are mentioned. Further research then revealed that of those approximately 6200 cases, 670—or about 11%—involved psychopharmacologic issues and concerns as important and significant elements of the case.

Using these data and this information, Table 10.2 gives a frequency distribution for these reported cases of psychopharmacologic mentions according to the area of the law in which they occur.

---

[1] <Footnote ID="Fn1"><Para ID="Par4">The bulk of the material in this chapter is drawn from an unpublished survey on "Applications of Psychopharmacology in the Law." Thanks go to Jeffrey Harris, Esquire, who conducted a good deal of the research for this survey.</Para></Footnote>

© The Author(s), under exclusive license to Springer Nature Switzerland AG 2022
D. P. Greenfield, *Psychopharmacology for Nonpsychiatrists*,
https://doi.org/10.1007/978-3-030-82507-2_10

Table 10.1 Applications of psychopharmacology to the law: an overview of reported cases by area of law

Area of the law	Applications and examples
Civil law	
Professional liability	Misrepresenting psychotropic medications
Personal injury	Psychiatric/neuropsychiatric damages (treatment aspects)
Product liability (medications)	Celebrex®; Fen-Fen® litigation
Employment law	Psychiatric/neuropsychiatric damages (treatment aspects)
Toxic torts	Psychiatric/neuropsychiatric damages (treatment aspects)
Mental health law	Psychiatric/neuropsychiatric damages (treatment aspects)
Regulatory law	Civil commitment (psychiatric patients and sexually violent predators/sexually dangerous persons); treatment issues
Testamentary/estate law	Competency to participate in bankruptcy preparation and proceedings
Other	Will contests (caveat proceedings)
Criminal law	
Psychiatric defenses	Legal insanity; diminished capacity (e.g., "Prozac® Defense"); intoxication; irresistible impulse; passion-provocation (mitigation)
Competency to proceed to trial; "Miranda" competency	Effects of psychotropic medications (e.g., "chemical sanity")
Others	
Family law	Effects of illicit drugs or psychotropic medications on children, adolescents, and adults

Table 10.2 Frequency distribution of reported cases by area of law

Area of law	Anti-agent	Illicit substance	Botanical, herbal, nutraceutical, and (dietary) supplement agent
Bankruptcy	1	0	1
Civil competency	5	0	0
Consumer fraud	1	0	8
Constitutional law/civil rights	20	11	6
Contract law (including health coverage)	13	1	1
Copyright/intellectual property/patent law	27	4	5
Criminal law	43	88	5
Defamation	0	2	0
Disability law (including Social Security)	73	8	1
Education law	5	1	0
False advertising	26	2	2
Family law	0	0	5
Mental health law	33	10	1
Negligence law	11	0	0
Personal injury	13	0	1
Product liability	9	4	6
Professional liability	57	0	8
Professional liability: malpractice	53	4	1
Regulation/administration	11	7	0
Unfair competition	0	0	3
Will contest (caveat proceeding)	11	0	3
Workers compensation	0	3	0

Conversely, Tables 10.3, 10.4, and 10.5 give frequency distributions for these reported cases of areas of the law according to the three broad categories of psychopharmacologic medications or drugs in which they occur:

- The "anti" class of medications (Table 10.3);
- Illicit drugs (Table 10.4); and.
- Botanical, herbal, nutraceutical, and (dietary) supplements agents (Table 10.5).

Table 10.3 Frequency distribution of reported cases by "anti" class of medication, high to low order

Anti-addiction	89
Anti-anxiety	67
Anti-depressant	67
Anti-psychotic	67
Anti-ADHD	36
Anti-pain (including fibromyalgia)	25
Anti-insomnia	22
Anti-appetite	19
Antiparkinsonian	17
Anti-convulsant	12
Anti-dementia	11
Anti-obsessive	9
Anti-sex	9
Anti-impotence	8
Anti-manic	8
Anti-pain	5
Anti-aggression	0

From a survey of "Anti-agents" using an earlier classification system

Table 10.4 Frequency distribution of reported cases by type of illicit drug

Stimulants	
Cocaine	14
Amphetamines/methamphetamines	21
Depressants	
Heroin	14
Opioids	16
Hallucinogens	
Marijuana/hashish	25
LSD	10
Mescaline	17
MDMA	13
PCP/ketamine	32
Ecstasy	12

Table 10.5 Frequency distribution of reported cases by type of botanical, herbal, nutraceutical, or (dietary) supplement agent, high to low order

Green tea	7	Kava kava	2
Aloe vera	5	Psyllium	2
Capsicum	5	Stevia	2
Ephedra (ma huang)	5	Arnica	1
Lycopene	5	Black cohosh	1
Magnesium	5	CoQ10	1
St. John's wort	5	Echinacea	1
Chamomile	4	Evening primrose	1
Lecithin	3	5-methylfolate	1
Milk thistle	3	Garlic	1
Fatty acid	3	Gotu kola	1
Selenium	3	Lemon balm	1
Siberian ginseng	3	Passion flower	1
Cranberry	2	Senna	1
Dong quai	2	Valerian root	1
Ginseng	2		

Given the wide range and number of reported legal cases significantly involving psychopharmacology in only this 10-year period, and recognizing that these reported cases represent only the "tip of the iceberg" of legal cases in which psycho-pharmacology plays a role, it behooves the legal professional to have at least a passing understanding of psychopharmacology. That is the purpose and goal of this part of this book: To present the busy legal professional with an easy-to-read, broad, not overly technical, user-friendly, concise, and convenient *Primer* of psychopharmacology to give the professional a practical passing understanding of this potentially daunting subject.

In addition, Chaps. 11 and 12 ("Selection and Use of Experts: Five Questions" and "Evaluating Versus Treating Doctor/Therapist: A Word to the Wise") present and discuss these two important topics in litigation, in the context of psychopharmacologic issues and concerns. "Forewarned is forearmed!"

A Note on References

Rather than burdening the reader with excessive and detailed references and citations in this *Primer*, given below are particularly useful selected references. In addition, other specific references and citations will be given in parentheses throughout the *Primer*. For further information and details about any topics presented and discussed in this book, the interested reader is referred not only to the following list of selected references but also to applicable textbooks, monographs, electronic databases, print articles and materials, internet sources, and other applicable resources.

Selected References

- Black DW, Andreasen NC. Introductory textbook of psychiatry. 6th ed. American Psychiatric Publishing, Inc.; 2014. (A solid basic textbook of psychiatry.)
- Multiple Authors. Diagnostic and statistical manual of mental health disorders (*DSM-5*). 5th ed. American Psychiatry Association, Inc.; 2013. (This book is the controversial "bible" for primarily American and Canadian psychiatric diagnoses.)
- The comparable international work to the *DSM-5* is currently the 2019 International Classification of Diseases (*ICD-10*). 10th ed. World Health Organization. (The *ICD-11* was due for adoption in 2020.)
- Frances A. Saving normal: an insider's revolt against out-of-control psychiatric diagnosis, big pharma, and the medicalization of ordinary life. Harper Collins Publishers: 2013. (The subtitle says it all! See Chap. 4 in this *Primer*.)
- Ghaemi SN. Clinical psychopharmacology: principles and practice. Oxford University Press: 2019. (A scholarly, detailed, and lengthy overview of psychopharmacology, also covering social practice and research/methodologic aspects of the field.)
- Hales RE, Yudofsky ST, Roberts LW, et al., editors. The American Psychiatric Publishing textbook of psychiatry. 6th ed. American Psychiatric Publishing, Inc.; 2014. (A standard, detailed encyclopedic textbook tome, for reference. A seventh edition is available, copyright 2019, with updated coverage in a number of areas.)
- Harrington A. Mind fixers: psychiatry's troubled search for the biology of mental illness. W.W. Norton and Company; 2019. (A historical and scholarly review of the topic, including some of the same topics as *Saving Normal* listed above.)
- Puzantian T, Carlat DJ. Medication fact book for psychiatric practice. 6th ed. Carlat Publishing, LLC; 2020. (A very useful "cookbook" for psychotropic prescribing, conveniently organized and presented for the practitioner.)
- Watters E. Crazy like us: the globalization of the American psyche. Free Press; 2010. (Psychiatric diagnostic issues similar to those in *Saving Normal*, with an international focus.)
- Weil A. Mind over meds: know when drugs are necessary, when alternatives are better—and when to let your body heal on its own. Little, Brown and Company; 2017. (A balanced and holistic approach to pharmacology and psychopharmacology by the popular "guru" of these fields.)

Selected Internet References

With the surfeit of internet resources, websites of all imaginable types and quality, and numerous related electronic sources of information and data, the reader, clinician, researcher, and member of the public—patient/client or not—may easily become confused about where to go and what to accept in learning psychopharmacology and psychopharmacotherapy. In this vein, a productive way to navigate the bewildering array of such sources consists of dividing them into several categories, viz.

1. Refereed ("peer-reviewed;" "juried") scientific, technical, and professional journals, newsletters, and the like, including e-journals, e-newsletters, and other open-source e-publications. Selected examples include:

   - *Journal of Clinical Psychopharmacology* (peer-reviewed independent professional journal)
   - *Experimental & Clinical Psychopharmacology* (peer-reviewed professional journal of the American Psychological Association)
   - *Journal of Psychopharmacology* (peer-reviewed professional journal of the British Association for Psychopharmacology)
   - *Psychopharmacology* (Berlin/Heidelberg; Springer Publications)

2. Government and academic/research institutions, publications and e-publications and associated websites. Selected examples include:

   - National Institute of Mental Health (NIMH) website, affiliated institutes, programs, centers, websites, and publications (electronic and print)
   - National Institute on Alcoholism and Alcohol Abuse (NIAAA) website, affiliated institutes, programs and centers, and websites and publications (electronic and print)
   - National Institute on Drug Abuse (NIDA) website, affiliated institutes, centers, programs and websites, and publications (electronic and print)
   - Canadian Centre on Substance Abuse (CCSA), affiliated programs and publications (electronic and print)
   - National Center on Addiction and Substance Abuse at Columbia University (NCASACU), programs and publications (electronic and print)

3. Journals, magazines, societies, and associated websites. Selected examples include:

   - *Psychology Today*
   - *Scientific American*
   - *Scientific American Mind*

As a practical matter, in researching particular topics electronically in psychopharmacology/psychopharmacotherapy, the logical rule—as with everything else—is to search for topic(s), keyword(s), and the like on a search engine, then to narrow the search with entries given by the search engine. An important factor to keep in mind here is the reliability, accuracy, and quality of the source: Sources from (1) and (2)—above—are considered more reliable than those in (3), generally. Those in (3), in turn, are generally considered more reliable than personal blogs, newsletters, product websites, company websites, and the like.

Chapter 11
Selection and Use of Experts: Five Questions

In "Alice's Adventures in Wonderland" (In Carroll L. *Lewis Carroll: The Complete Illustrated Works*. Gramercy Books; 1982), the Queen's response to the King's instructions to "Let the jury consider their verdict..." was "No, no! Sentence first, verdict afterwards."

Analogously, the prospective expert witness's response to counsel's (and sometimes to the court's) request for "a report addressing such-and-such" should be "Don't you want to know my opinion before you get my report?" This unsubtle response by the expert demonstrates the fundamental **difference in advocacy** between attorneys and their experts:

- Attorneys are zealous advocates for their **clients**, whereas.
- The attorneys'/courts' **experts** are zealous advocates for their opinions about the attorneys'/courts' **questions** about the clients.

With this basic and important distinction in mind, this chapter will next present and discuss "Selection and Use of Experts: Five Questions."

The logical first question for the reader of this chapter is "Do I need an expert?"

The second question is "What type of expert do I need for my case, for whatever reason I might need that expert?" The second question, convoluted though it may seem, suggests several underlying sub-questions. The sub-questions are:

1. Do I actually need an expert? Why?
2. If yes, what type of expert do I need?
3. In the area of psychopharmacology, what type of experts are available?
4. As an extension of Question 3: Do I need an expert who can, and actually has, prescribed these psychotropic drugs or medications? And if yes, how do I go about selecting that expert?
5. Can or should my expert do more (or less) than evaluate, offer an opinion, and testify in a case?

© The Author(s), under exclusive license to Springer Nature
Switzerland AG 2022
D. P. Greenfield, *Psychopharmacology for Nonpsychiatrists*,
https://doi.org/10.1007/978-3-030-82507-2_11

This chapter will address each of these questions in turn, in a practical and common sense way. The chapter will also address questions and concerns from the expert's perspective about the litigation process.

Question 1. Do I actually need an expert? Why?

General legal requirements for use of experts are discussed in relation to Table 11.1. Without reiterating the formal statutory or legal/evidentiary requirements for the use of experts in the law, and skipping first to the broader perspective of practicality, we are aware that in our increasingly complex and technical world, knowledge is vital and expertise is crucial. When properly used, evidence offered by a qualified expert in a forensic setting—hearing, trial, deposition—as a negotiating tool, in a practical context, or in any other such way, may be a key to an attorney's successful representation of their client (see Table 11.2).

Table 11.1 Ways of using experts in legal/forensic matters

Educating retaining counsel in the area of the expert's expertise.
Advising counsel about strengths and weaknesses of the case from the expert's perspective.
Providing counsel with information and opinions about opposing expert(s), when applicable and when possible.
Reviewing available records and materials about a case and consulting with retaining counsel **before issuing a written report**.
Consulting and discussing all aspects of a case with retaining counsel throughout the litigation process.
Working with retaining counsel in any other appropriate and acceptable way.

Table 11.2 Criminal and civil issues in which mental health experts may be used

Traditional criminal responsibility-reducing psychiatric defenses	Future dangerousness
Legal insanity	Miranda (constitutional rights) waiver
Diminished capacity	Mitigation of penalty (federal sentencing guidelines)
Intoxication	Suicide
Irresistible impulse	Transfer (waiver; referral issues for juveniles)
Sex offenses	**Employment law** (sexual harassment; discrimination; others)
Sex offenses	**Personal injury** (including sexual abuse)
Sexually violent predators (SVPs) and sexually dangerous persons (SDPs)	**Professional liability** (malpractice)
Community notification (Megan's Law registrants)	**Mental health law** (civil commitment, including sexually violent predators (SVPs) and sexually deviant predators (SDPs)
Domestic violence	**Toxic exposure**
Malingering	**Professional regulation**
Arson	**Will contests**
Competency to stand (proceed to) trial	**Dram-shop liability**
Mitigation issues (death penalty)	**Competency** (civil)
Embezzlement	**Divorce**
Battered woman (spouse) syndrome (syndrome evidence cases)	**Custody and visitation**
Elder abuse	

Adapted from Greenfield and Gottschalk (2009)

A series of cases beginning in 1923 (see Table 11.3) broadened the acceptability of scientific forensic experts considerably, making way for many different types of forensic "experts." In the legal context, a stricter interpretation of the words "expert evidence," "opinion evidence," and "forensic expert" suggests that any type of expert input can assist the court in a resolution of a question or issue.[1] The legal system has become increasingly dependent on experts providing their factual and opinion evidence in fields ranging throughout the alphabet from "Accounting" to "Zoology."

Table 11.3 Summary of salient evidentiary features for expert testimony

Frye v. United States 293 F. 1013 (D.C. Circuit, 1923)	Daubert v. Merrell Dow 509 U.S. 579, L.S. 4805 113 S. Ct. 2786 (1993)	Kumho Tire Co. v. Carmichael 526 U.S. 137 119 S. Ct. 1167 (1999)
The "general acceptance" rule	Is it testable, and has it been tested? Has it been subjected to peer review and publication? In the case of a particular scientific technique, what is the known or potential rate of error? What (if any) are the standards that control the techniques operation? To what extent is the theory accepted in the scientific community (the "general acceptance" rule)?	Expert testimony not based only on "scientific" knowledge may be accepted as evidence in court

---

[1] The legal community has come a long way since the first recorded use, in 1783, of forensic evidence and expert opinion.

In addition to the traditional ways in which experts are used in litigation, several less discussed but equally important uses of experts ought to be kept in mind by attorneys. These include educating counsel in the area of the expert's field; advising counsel about strengths and weaknesses of the case from the expert's perspective; providing counsel with information and opinions about the opposing expert(s) when possible and applicable; reviewing available records and materials about a case (including the opposing expert's written report, if available) and consulting with counsel before issuing a written report; consulting with counsel and discussing with counsel all applicable aspects of a case throughout the litigation process; and working with counsel in any other appropriate and acceptable way that counsel sees fit.

Of course, the opposite is true of the need for counsel to work closely with the expert they have hired, including providing, in a timely manner, all essential materials and documents for the expert to review; making time and being available to discuss all applicable aspects of the case with the expert; and otherwise aiding the expert in any other appropriate ways.

In the real world, such factors pertaining to prospective experts as expense, availability, quality and reputation, cooperativeness, and so forth will influence the attorney's decision about whether to retain an expert.

However, as a practical matter, the applicability of a variant of the well-known attorney's "smell test" ("If it doesn't smell right, it probably isn't.") will likely be useful for deciding whether to retain an expert for any given case: "If it smells like I need an expert for this case, I probably do." And merely because the expert does not, in the end, testify in the case does not mean that the expert was not needed on the case.

Question 2. If yes, what type of expert do I need?
Having made the decision that an expert is needed for a case, for whatever reason, this second question must be addressed: What type of expert do I need?

Dividing the predominant areas of the law for present purposes into criminal law, civil law, and family law, one can list the types of experts most frequently used within each area, as noted below.

- In criminal matters, frequently encountered forensic expertise will come through medical, mental health, dental, accident reconstruction, fingerprint, DNA, ballistics, computer science, and other related such experts, to address such questions as the cause and timing of death or injury, identification of victims, and others.
- In civil matters, because of the wide variety of substantive aspects of cases, a great variety of questions to be addressed by experts will be encountered. This variety may include virtually any question brought out in a civil matter: Accident specialists, forensic accountants, engineers, and many other types of traditional and non-traditional experts may be relevant. As an example of the wide range of types of cases in which one particular forensic expert—the mental health expert—might be used, Table 11.2, adapted from *Writing Forensic Reports* (Greenfield DP, Gottschalk J. *Writing Forensic Reports: A Guide for Mental*

Health Professionals. Springer; 2009), gives examples of the types of cases in which mental health experts may be utilized.

- In family law, in this author's experience, mental health experts are the most widely used, to assist the court in resolving such concerns as child custody (and the best interest of the child); fair treatment of a spouse or partner with mental illness of some sort (and often on psychotropic medications); and other such examples.

As every law student knows, for purposes of using an expert in litigation, it is not sufficient simply to have an "expert" carry on in court only with the idea of somehow "educating the jury," or about expressing an opinion about this or that pet theory: "Junk science in the courtroom" is not allowed, and court standards for the admissibility of expert evidence must be met. The standards most often applied, in this writer's experience, are the *Frye* standard from 1923 and the more recent *Daubert/Kumho Tire Co.*1999 decision, and their progeny, beginning in 1993. Table 11.3 outlines the salient features of these two standards. The *Frye* and *Daubert* standards generally refer to the admissibility of expert evidence of any type— including written expert reports—and apply in both state and federal jurisdictions. However, some states use the *Frye* standard, some use the *Daubert* and progeny standard, and some use both (such as New Jersey, as of this writing, criminal cases require the *Frye* standard for experts, and civil cases require the *Daubert* standard).

It behooves counsel to advise the expert which standard applies for any given case, and it behooves the expert to know or to find out that applicable standard.

Question 3. In the area of psychopharmacology, what types of experts are available?

Having made the decision that an expert is needed for a particular case and that the case involves drugs, medications, toxicologic agents, botanicals/herbals-nutraceuticals/(dietary) supplements—in other words, any of the substances discussed in Part 1, "Psychopharmacology," of this book—**how** do I decide what specific type of expert I need? and **what** types of experts in these areas are available? These issues will be discussed next.

To begin, retaining counsel has to **find**, **select**, and **retain** an expert.

Finding an expert, first of all, implies that the attorney knows the type of expert needed. In psychopharmacologic and related cases, this usually boils down to physicians, toxicologists, clinical pharmacologists, nurse practitioners, physician assistants, and other professionals whose main area of expertise involves study, teaching, research, and/or prescribing psychotropic agents, or combinations of these activities. Two additional principles apply here:

1. In cases in which opposing counsel has already retained an expert, especially in situations involving clinical practice issues, an expert of at least the same or a comparable discipline ought to be selected, especially in potential jury trial situations. This principle of "like begets like" generally applies to selection of experts by counsel, in my experience. For example, a practicing psychologist licensed to prescribe in New Mexico (see Chap. 3) pitted against another such

psychologist would create an "even playing field," all other factors being equal. However, such a psychologist pitted against an academic practicing physician/ clinical psychopharmacologist would likely be perceived, especially by a jury, as "outclassed," regardless of the quality of the psychologist's expertise and ability to testify persuasively and compellingly.

Other considerations exist, such as whether to select a local or out-of-town expert; whether to select an experienced forensic expert—a "litigation consul- tant"—or an experienced clinical or academic expert without considerable liti- gation experience; and other such factors. These must necessarily be decided on a case-by-case basis.

2. In addition to the "like begets like" principle (above) of expert selection, counsel needs to know what types of experts are potentially available with expertise in psychopharmacology and related areas. As a practical matter, such an expert will often be found in the mental health profession, as well as in the scientific disci- plines of pharmacology and toxicology and their forensic subdivisions. The interested reader is referred to applicable books, monographs, electronic databases, internet sources, and the like, recognizing that not all types of mental health professionals discussed in this volume prescribe medications or deal extensively with psychopharmacology.

Next comes **selecting** an expert, once the type of expert has been identified. While an extensive discussion of all of the factors which might enter into selection criteria for an expert is well beyond the scope of this book, some basic and practical points should be considered. Among such factors are whether to select an expert experienced in litigation **or** an experienced academic practitioner with little court- room presence (to name one such dichotomy); whether to select an out-of-town expert without ties to the professional and/or legal community in which the litiga- tion takes place **or** a local expert (presumably with those ties); whether to select the treating professional of a litigant (which I strongly do **not** recommend: See Chap. 12); whether to select a highly reputed "superstar" expert whom counsel does not know; and other relevant common sense considerations.

To begin the search process for an expert, counsel is well advised to consult with colleagues in the legal community for referrals. In that way, prospective experts will have already been vetted to some extent. Failing in that approach or wanting to expand the search, counsel could consult with any number of professional societies (e.g., medical and medical specialty societies) whose members provide forensic expert consultation services. Access to these sources can be either through the inter- net or through print resources. Directories and forensic consulting services specifi- cally designed to provide expert referrals for attorneys may be consulted, such as those listed in a number of publications like the state-based *Lawyers' Diary* directo- ries, some of which are affiliated with state and national bar associations and legal specialty societies.

The final step in the process of counsel's selecting an expert witness is the **reten- tion** of the expert. This step assumes that the proposed expert meets all of the neces- sary professional qualifications and that from the interpersonal perspective, retaining counsel and the proposed expert can work together. The litigation process tends to strain both nerves and relationships. Prior to actual retention, counsel should interview their prospective expert both to discuss substantive aspects of the case at hand and to screen the expert for psychological compatibility and ease of interpersonal communication. Once the decision to retain is made, a formal written contractual agreement should be entered into with the expert, which specifies terms, conditions, scheduling issues, financial arrangements, and other such aspects of the attorney–expert relationship. Sometimes attorneys will promulgate such a document; sometimes experts use their own; and sometimes expert consultation services use contracts involving all three entities (i.e., the retaining attorney, the expert, and the service). In any event, before the actual work by the expert begins, the terms, conditions, and requirements of the expert's consultation should be as clear as possible to all concerned, to facilitate the working relationship between counsel and the expert.

In private sector cases, the expert is ultimately paid by the attorney's client, albeit indirectly. Since the expert forensic services provided are not clinical consultation, evaluation, or treatment in nature but rather are consultative services **to** the client's attorney **about** the attorney's client, payment to the expert should be made by the attorney, through the attorney's client trust or escrow account (this type of account has a variety of names), directly to the expert, from monies paid to the attorney by the attorney's client with funds earmarked for costs associated with litigation. With that practice, no question of a doctor–patient, psychologist–client, social worker/counselor–client relationship or other such therapist–client treatment relationship would arise. In public sector cases, the expert is usually paid directly by the retaining agency. However, that agency may have arrangements with its clients in which the clients pay some or all of the costs of representation and litigation (such as the Office of the Public Defender in New Jersey, which charges non-indigent clients an initial administrative fee and a subsequent hourly rate for attorneys' and related services). Experts are generally not paid by attorneys' clients in the public sector (such as Public Defender and Attorney General cases) or quasi-public agencies (such as legal aid organizations).

Volumes[2] could be written about the relationship between counsel and expert once the expert's consultation has begun. Without belaboring the obvious and acknowledging that this relationship can be difficult for both, especially during trial (or hearing, or deposition), four salient features deserve emphasis:

- The first is **communication**. Counsel and their experts should ascertain their preferred mode of communication (i.e., telephone, email, fax, texting, or a combination of these) and should maintain frequent communication with each other—virtually constant during trial (or hearing, or deposition)—through that mode. As any frustrated attorney or expert will confirm, violation of this rule will

---

[2] *For a not-too-serious treatment of these issues,* see: Greenfield DP. *A Practical Guide to Forensic Mental Health Consultation Through Aphorisms and Caveats.* Cognella Academic Publishing; In Press.

be at least troublesome and even infuriating for either counsel, the expert, or both, and at worst, may jeopardize the outcome of the case.

- The second is **preparation**. As in any phase of the litigation process, the importance of thorough mutual preparation (by telephone, electronic contact, or in person, although the last is usually preferable) by counsel and expert cannot be underestimated.
- The third is **consistency**. The ups and downs of litigation can be very trying for both counsel and their experts, and both may be pressed to depart from previously agreed upon parameters and elements of the arrangements between them. This is not advisable, in my experience, no matter what the exigencies of the litigation process may be.
- The fourth is **flexibility**. This is especially illustrated by the situation presented by the current COVID-19 pandemic, in which virtual communication is necessitated by social distancing requirements, whether or not the attorneys, experts, and/or parties to litigation like that practice.

Question 4. Do I need an expert who can, and actually has, prescribed psychotropic drugs or medications? And if yes, how do I go about selecting that expert?

A response to this question clearly should be based on the nature of the case for which the expert is sought and may be considered an extension of the "like begets like" principle articulated earlier in this chapter. For example, in civil malpractice matters involving psychotropic drugs or medications, an expert—such as a practicing physician—who can opine about prescribing from personal, professional experience would generally be preferable to one who has not.

On the other hand, in a product liability case involving complex statistical and technical analysis, such consultation might be beyond the ability of a professional who is predominantly a clinical practitioner. In that example, an academic or industry-based expert would likely be preferable. Decisions of this type need to be made on a case-by-case basis, with retaining counsel aware of the professional capabilities, licensing authority, and experience of potential expert witnesses. Locating such experts follows the same principles discussed earlier in this chapter: Word-of-mouth recommendations, directories, previous experience and contact with the proposed expert, professional societies, academic institutions, industry settings, the internet, and other such referral sources.

Question 5. Can or should my expert do more (or less) than evaluate, offer an opinion, and testify in a case?

Although any forensic expert's advocacy position—to develop and offer an expert opinion about someone of concern being evaluated, and to be an advocate for that opinion, not for the person or the concern evaluated—in a case is different from the retaining attorney's position (to be an advocate for their client, who is evaluated by the forensic expert), the expert may legitimately be called upon to do more in any given case than simply evaluate an attorney's client, develop, and write an opinion about the forensic issues in the case at hand and testify about that opinion (when testimony occurs). Table 11.1 alludes to this expanded view of the role of a forensic expert, especially in terms of the last two bullet points ("…consulting with counsel and discussing with counsel all applicable aspects of a case throughout the litigation process; and working with counsel in any other appropriate and acceptable way that counsel sees fit...").

As a practical matter, in my view, no expert should agree to consult on a case without being willing to testify at trial, deposition, and/or hearing about their opinion in that case. Conversely, no attorney should expect that their retained expert will only consult and assist in a case short of (and not including) testifying in this case. While most cases in litigation do not go to trial, the retaining attorney and retained expert generally ought to assume that any given case will go to trial (and/or hearing, and/or deposition), and should prepare accordingly, intensively or thoroughly: "It comes with the territory." Once a trial (and/or deposition, and/or hearing) is scheduled and likely to proceed, preparation begins. This process is described from the expert's perspective earlier in this chapter, and its importance cannot be overstated. One particular point in this context which should be emphasized is the usefulness of the expert's written report as a guide, or "trial notebook" for their testimony. This is a point discussed in detail in *Writing Forensic Reports: A Guide for Mental Health Professionals* (p. 179 of that book).

In addition to thorough preparation and knowledge of the expert's report, both personal and professional characteristics are necessary to present persuasive and convincing testimony in court, at a hearing, or at a deposition. It goes without saying that the testifying expert should dress carefully and conservatively, but not overdress. The expert should speak slowly and deliberately, making "bullet points" on direct examination which have been previously discussed and agreed upon by retaining counsel and making them in such a way as not to be an advocate for retaining counsel's client: Again, the advocacy position of representing counsel is **for** their client, whereas the advocacy position of the retained expert mental professional is **about** the retaining attorney's client.

In testifying, the expert should use clear, understandable, and straightforward language; present a friendly and informal—and not arrogant or distantly professional—demeanor; speak directly to the jury (in jury trials); present testimony in a conversational and story-telling style in easily understood words and terms; and not "speak down" to the court or the jury, no matter how technical or complicated the testimony content may be. All of these points should be made to or known by the expert during preparation for direct examination testimony, and the mental health expert in their expanded role, as described above, should point out strengths and weaknesses in their opinion and testimony, as relevant to the case.

All of the above are points relating to strategy which the mental health expert in this expanded role should discuss with retaining counsel. Conversely, these are also strategic points which retaining counsel should expect from their retained expert in that expert's expanded role.

Professional literature abounds with discussions and advice about the use of mental health expert witnesses, but space limitations do not permit a comprehensive review of this broad topic. The foregoing points, in broad strokes, have been particularly practical and helpful to this author over the years of his forensic psychiatric practice.

Liability of Experts

This next section shifts from the lawyer's perspective to the expert's perspective. Aside from feeling the stresses and strains of deadlines, testimony, and the myriad of other potential problems generated for the forensic expert consultant in litigation, two questions at the back of any expert's mind are: (1) "Can I get into trouble from performing this expert witness work?" and (2) "If I do, what kind of trouble will that be?" In my experience, this is especially the case with mental health and other clinicians—licensed and regulated practitioners, generally, of any mental health or other medical or related professional who treats patients/clients, in a formal doctor–patient, or therapist–client relationship—who are not acting in that capacity in performing forensic evaluations. Whether those clinicians are private practitioners, full- or part-time academics, hospital or other institutional employees, or in any other occupational or professional setting does not matter for these concerns. The specter of being sued, whether for clinical treatment or forensic consultation, is disturbing for any clinician or practitioner.

The response to the first question ("Can I get into trouble from performing this expert witness work?") is simple and straightforward: "Yes. Anything is possible." Without belaboring the obvious to a legal audience, in tort law, virtually any person can be sued at any time for any reason at all. The more important question is whether a potential civil suit against a forensic expert witness has standing and merit and whether its basis is sound and likely to succeed against the expert.

The answer to the first question leads inexorably to the second: "What kind of trouble will that be?" In other words, what are the potential sources of liability for the forensic expert witness? While commentators agree that the traditional doctor–patient treatment relationship does not apply for the evaluating/consulting forensic expert, some requirements in the forensic expert–evaluee relationship do apply. In "Liability of the Forensic Psychiatrist," for example, Willick et al., describe the following conceptual framework (Table 11.4) for identifying sources of liability of forensic experts, then present a series of examples which illustrate the framework, specifically for forensic psychiatric experts. (Willick D, et al. Liability of the forensic psychiatrist. In: Rosner R, editor. *Principles and Practice of Forensic Psychiatry.* 2nd ed. Taylor & Francis Group; 2009).

Table 11.4 Forensic consultation

1. **Who** is the forensic client?
2. **What** task is being performed?
3. Is the task being performed with **legal protections** such as pursuant to a court order?

Adapted from Willick et al. (2009)

Some examples of forensic liability, given by Willick et al., are based on claims of **negligence**, **intentional torts**, and **federal civil rights actions**.

As a practical matter, in the medical context, even though forensic third party evaluations are not the same as consultations/evaluations in the treatment of patients, "…The law considers both third-party evaluations and evaluations conducted for treatment purposes to constitute the practice of medicine… case law does not differentiate between them…" and a limited physician–patient relationship has been articulated concerning duties of physicians (experts) toward third-party evaluees. (Gold L, Davidson J. Do you understand your risk? Liability and third-party evaluations in civil litigations. *The Journal of the American Academy of Psychiatry and the Law*. AAPL. 2007).

A final area of potential liability and risk for forensic experts lies in alleged violations of applicable practice (e.g., medical, for physician) law and regulations, ethical codes, and practice guidelines. Actions in these areas may not directly or inexorably lead to civil lawsuits, but they may lead to disciplinary actions or censure by the expert's legal licensing, registration, and regulatory agencies; professional societies; specialty certification boards; or other such actions. One particular area of concern in this regard pertains to healthcare professionals who engage in forensic activities in jurisdictions in which they are not licensed in their health profession.

In addition to the customary protections for any forensic expert practitioner— such as having adequate professional liability insurance, having a clear and written understanding with retaining counsel about the parameters and requirements of the forensic consultations (as also discussed above), having the forensic work done pursuant to court order (with resulting quasi-judicial immunity) when possible, and having a written confidentiality disclosure consent statement for each evaluation—a practical rule-of-thumb defining professional malpractice (professional liability) for the forensic expert consultant may be seen as a modification of the "Four Ds" in tort law ("Duty" to treat; "Dereliction" in the "Duty," resulting in; "Damages" to the client, proximately or; "Directly" caused by the "Dereliction") which constitutes clinical malpractice: The forensic expert has a:

- "Duty" to apply the best scientific bases to their evaluation of the third-party evaluee;

> but

- If "Derelict" in that "Duty," resulting in
- "Damages" to counsel's case, there must be a proximate,

> or

- "Direct" relationship between the "Duty" and the "Damages."

In this vein, for forensic medical experts, some protection from potential legal liability for consultations in which opinions are ultimately determined to be erroneous or inadmissible is found in endorsement of the concept that experts not be held liable for such opinions as long as the opinions were based on a proper, sound, and scientific evaluation.

In this chapter, and as described in the Author's Disclaimer Note (located near the beginning of this book), the information given in the three forensic/legal chapters of this *Primer* should not be construed or taken as legal advice, which as a non-lawyer or legal professional, the author is not competent to give, and which can be given only by an attorney or qualified legal professional.

A Note on References

Rather than burdening the reader with excessive and detailed references and citations in this *Primer*, given below are particularly useful selected references. In addition, other specific references and citations will be given in parentheses throughout the *Primer*. For further information and details about any topics presented and discussed in this book, the interested reader is referred not only to the following list of selected references but also to applicable textbooks, monographs, electronic databases, print articles and materials, internet sources, and other applicable resources.

Selected References

- Black DW, Andreasen NC. Introductory textbook of psychiatry. 6th ed. American Psychiatric Publishing, Inc.; 2014. (A solid basic textbook of psychiatry.)
- Multiple Authors. Diagnostic and statistical manual of mental health disorders (*DSM-5*). 5th ed. American Psychiatry Association, Inc.; 2013. (This book is the controversial "bible" for primarily American and Canadian psychiatric diagnoses.)
- The comparable international work to the *DSM-5* is currently the 2019 International classification of diseases (*ICD-10*). 10th ed. World Health Organization. (The *ICD-11* was due for adoption in 2020.)
- Frances A. Saving normal: an insider's revolt against out-of-control psychiatric diagnosis, big pharma, and the medicalization of ordinary life. Harper Collins Publishers; 2013. (The subtitle says it all! See Chap. 4 in this *Primer*.)
- Ghaemi SN. Clinical psychopharmacology: principles and practice. Oxford University Press; 2019. (A scholarly, detailed, and lengthy overview of psycho-pharmacology, also covering social practice and research/methodologic aspects of the field.)
- Hales RE, Yudofsky ST, Roberts LW, editors, et al. The American Psychiatric Publishing textbook of psychiatry. 6th ed. American Psychiatric Publishing, Inc.; 2014. (A standard, detailed encyclopedic textbook tome, for reference. A seventh edition is available, copyright 2019, with updated coverage in a number of areas.)
- Harrington A. Mind fixers: psychiatry's troubled search for the biology of mental illness. W.W. Norton and Company; 2019. (A historical and scholarly review of the topic, including some of the same topics as *Saving Normal* listed above.)

- Puzantian T, Carlat DJ. Medication fact book for psychiatric practice. 6th ed. Carlat Publishing, LLC; 2020. (A very useful "cookbook" for psychotropic prescribing, conveniently organized and presented for the practitioner.)
- Watters E. Crazy like us: the globalization of the American psyche. Free Press; 2010. (Psychiatric diagnostic issues similar to those in *Saving Normal*, with an international focus.)
- Weil A. Mind over meds: know when drugs are necessary, when alternatives are better—and when to let your body heal on its own. Little, Brown and Company; 2017. (A balanced and holistic approach to pharmacology and psychopharmacology by the popular "guru" of these fields.)

Selected Internet References

With the surfeit of internet resources, websites of all imaginable types and quality, and numerous related electronic sources of information and data, the reader, clinician, researcher, and member of the public—patient/client or not—may easily become confused about where to go and what to accept in learning psychopharmacology and psychopharmacotherapy. In this vein, a productive way to navigate the bewildering array of such sources consists of dividing them into several categories, viz.

1. Referreed ("peer-reviewed;" "juried") scientific, technical, and professional journals, newsletters, and the like, including e-journals, e-newsletters, and other open-source e-publications. Selected examples include:

   - *Journal of Clinical Psychopharmacology* (peer-reviewed independent professional journal)
   - *Experimental & Clinical Psychopharmacology* (peer-reviewed professional journal of the American Psychological Association)
   - *Journal of Psychopharmacology* (peer-reviewed professional journal of the British Association for Psychopharmacology)
   - *Psychopharmacology* (Berlin/Heidelberg; Springer Publications)

2. Government and academic/research institutions, publications and e-publications and associated websites. Selected examples include:

   - National Institute of Mental Health (NIMH) website, affiliated institutes, programs, centers, websites, and publications (electronic and print)
   - National Institute on Alcoholism and Alcohol Abuse (NIAAA) website, affiliated institutes, programs and centers, and websites and publications (electronic and print)
   - National Institute on Drug Abuse (NIDA) website, affiliated institutes, centers, programs and websites, and publications (electronic and print)
   - Canadian Centre on Substance Abuse (CCSA), affiliated programs and publications (electronic and print)

- National Center on Addiction and Substance Abuse at Columbia University (NCASACU), programs and publications (electronic and print)

3. Journals, magazines, societies, and associated websites. Selected examples include:

- *Psychology Today*
- *Scientific American*
- *Scientific American Mind*

As a practical matter, in researching particular topics electronically in psychopharmacology/psychopharmacotherapy, the logical rule—as with everything else—is to search for topic(s), keyword(s), and the like on a search engine, then to narrow the search with entries given by the search engine. An important factor to keep in mind here is the reliability, accuracy, and quality of the source: Sources from (1) and (2)—above—are considered more reliable than those in (3), generally. Those in (3), in turn, are generally considered more reliable than personal blogs, newsletters, product websites, company websites, and the like.

Chapter 12
Evaluating Versus Treating Doctor/Therapist: A Word to the Wise

The reader of this *Primer* of primarily psychopharmacology/psychopharmacotherapy might well ask why this chapter is included in this book. One response to that question, as stated in the Preface, is that part of the intended audience for this book is the legal professional who interacts with psychopharmacology/psychopharmacotherapy in various ways, including litigation. But the other response, more geared to the overall readership of this book, is that prescribers—regardless of discipline, orientation, or professional qualifications—may be called upon, sometimes involuntarily, or at least unwillingly, to testify about their patients/clients as an expert witness, as a fact, or material witness (i.e., the "treating professional"), or as both, a hybrid of the treating professional with "expertise in the field" (as a trial attorney told me a number of years ago). This chapter will provide basic and practical information about this question.

But what is the bottom line answer to the conundrum posed by the title of this chapter? This writer's response—my word to the wise—in that regard, is a resounding "no," to employing the forensic services of a treating doctor/therapist for reasons to be presented and discussed below.

In the litigation context, prescribers of all disciplines and professions can serve as witnesses concerning patients/clients in two ways, viz., (1) as fact, or material witnesses, providing clinical information and testimony about their treatment of their own patients/clients and (2) as expert, or opinion witnesses, providing evidence and testimony about others evaluated by them for litigation purposes, who are not their own patients/clients.

That treating (prescribing, for present purposes) healthcare professionals ought to and do have a duty to provide the first service (i.e., as a fact, or material/treating witness) is mandated by legal (case law) precedents and by codes of ethics and professional conduct in a number of professional organizations (such as the APA and the AMA), in this writer's experience.

© The Author(s), under exclusive license to Springer Nature   163
Switzerland AG 2022
D. P. Greenfield, *Psychopharmacology for Nonpsychiatrists*,
https://doi.org/10.1007/978-3-030-82507-2_12

However, conflict in this area between legal/forensic practices (such as litigation and testimony) and clinical guidelines and sensibilities (such as confidentiality/privacy/privilege) necessarily arises in situations in which the boundary is blurred between the prescribing healthcare professional as treatment provider for a patient/client in litigation and that same professional as an opinion evidence "provider" (i.e., expert witness) for that same patient/client. Although the advisability of a clinician's serving as their patient's/client's expert witness remains controversial for some practitioners (legal **and** clinical), in this author's experience, that role on the part of the clinician presents a difficult role conflict for the clinician. That conflict is the bedrock contraindication to a clinician's serving as their patient's/client's expert witness. Concisely put, the treating clinician cannot objectively and with neutrality give opinion evidence about their patient/client (for whom the clinician is an advocate), especially if such opinion evidence disadvantages (i.e., does not advocate for) their client.

The following tables respectively give further reasons **for** (Table 12.1 "Pros") and **against** (Table 12.2 "Cons") treating clinicians' serving as experts for their patients/clients.

Table 12.1 "Pros:" reasons for the treating clinician to serve as expert witness

The treating clinician has had longer and more extensive contact with the patient/client/litigant and "knows" the patient/client better than an evaluating forensic clinician
The treating clinician would be less expensive to employ as forensic expert than would be an independent outside evaluating clinician
The treating clinician would be more invested as an advocate in the patient's/client's/litigant's legal matter than would be a neutral objective evaluating clinician
The practicing treating clinician might have more clinical experience—and therefore more credibility—than an outside evaluating clinician

Table 12.2 "Cons:" reasons for the treating clinician not to serve as expert witness (but for the evaluating clinician to serve as expert)

The outside evaluating clinician is *not* an advocate for the patient/client/litigant and can be unbiased and objective in their evaluation and opinion
The outside evaluating clinician does not have an ongoing relationship and/or financial interest in the outcome of the patient's/client's/litigant's legal matter
The outside evaluating clinician will more likely have greater experience and credibility in forensic evaluations than the treating clinician

Additional reasons and justifications both for and against treating clinicians' serving as expert witnesses for their patients/clients can be marshaled, including arguments pertaining to patient/client advocacy; psychodynamic and psychotherapeutic conflicts; financial considerations and interests in the outcome of a legal matter; and treating clinician bias (i.e., advocacy).

In the final analysis, this writer is not aware of any formal or informal prohibition against treating clinicians serving as forensic expert witnesses for their patients/clients. However, in view of the "pro" and "con" points and other such arguments presented and discussed in this chapter about that practice, the bottom line, or balance, requires that treating mental health professionals must be advocates for their patients/clients, as attorneys **must** be for their clients. To ask such clinicians to do otherwise by serving as a patient's/client's expert witness as well as that patient's/client's therapist is fraught with potential biases and conflicts, and thus should be avoided. A cautionary tale is raised by common sense and professional guidelines in this practice: "A word to the wise."

A Note on References

Rather than burdening the reader with excessive and detailed references and citations in this *Primer*, given below are particularly useful selected references. In addition, other specific references and citations will be given in parentheses throughout the *Primer*. For further information and details about any topics presented and discussed in this book, the interested reader is referred not only to the following list of selected references but also to applicable textbooks, monographs, electronic databases, print articles and materials, internet sources, and other applicable resources.

Selected References

- Black DW, Andreasen NC. Introductory textbook of psychiatry. 6th ed. American Psychiatric Publishing, Inc.; 2014. (A solid basic textbook of psychiatry.)
- Multiple Authors. Diagnostic and statistical manual of mental health disorders (*DSM-5*). 5th ed. American Psychiatry Association, Inc.; 2013. (This book is the controversial "bible" for primarily American and Canadian psychiatric diagnoses.)
- The comparable international work to the *DSM-5* is currently the 2019 International classification of diseases (*ICD-10*). 10th ed. World Health Organization. (The *ICD-11* was due for adoption in 2020.)
- Frances A. Saving normal: an insider's revolt against out-of-control psychiatric diagnosis, big pharma, and the medicalization of ordinary life. Harper Collins Publishers; 2013. (The subtitle says it all! See Chap. 4 in this *Primer*.)

- Ghaemi SN. Clinical psychopharmacology: principles and practice. Oxford University Press; 2019. (A scholarly, detailed, and lengthy overview of psychopharmacology, also covering social practice and research/methodologic aspects of the field.)
- Hales RE, Yudofsky ST, Roberts LW, editors, et al. The American Psychiatric Publishing textbook of psychiatry. 6th ed. American Psychiatric Publishing, Inc.; 2014. (A standard, detailed encyclopedic textbook tome, for reference. A seventh edition is available, copyright 2019, with updated coverage in a number of areas.)
- Harrington A. Mind fixers: psychiatry's troubled search for the biology of mental illness. W.W. Norton and Company; 2019. (A historical and scholarly review of the topic, including some of the same topics as *Saving Normal* listed above.)
- Puzantian T, Carlat DJ. Medication fact book for psychiatric practice. 6th ed. Carlat Publishing, LLC; 2020. (A very useful "cookbook" for psychotropic prescribing, conveniently organized and presented for the practitioner.)
- Watters E. Crazy like us: the globalization of the American psyche. Free Press; 2010. (Psychiatric diagnostic issues similar to those in *Saving Normal*, with an international focus.)
- Weil A. Mind over meds: know when drugs are necessary, when alternatives are better—and when to let your body heal on its own. Little, Brown and Company; 2017. (A balanced and holistic approach to pharmacology and psychopharmacology by the popular "guru" of these fields.)

Selected Internet References

With the surfeit of internet resources, websites of all imaginable types and quality, and numerous related electronic sources of information and data, the reader, clinician, researcher, and member of the public—patient/client or not—may easily become confused about where to go and what to accept in learning psychopharmacology and psychopharmacotherapy. In this vein, a productive way to navigate the bewildering array of such sources consists of dividing them into several categories, viz.

1. Referreed ("peer-reviewed;" "juried") scientific, technical, and professional journals, newsletters, and the like, including e-journals, e-newsletters, and other open-source e-publications. Selected examples include:

   - *Journal of Clinical Psychopharmacology* (peer-reviewed independent professional journal)
   - *Experimental & Clinical Psychopharmacology* (peer-reviewed professional journal of the American Psychological Association)
   - *Journal of Psychopharmacology* (peer-reviewed professional journal of the British Association for Psychopharmacology)
   - *Psychopharmacology* (Berlin/Heidelberg; Springer Publications)

2. Government and academic/research institutions, publications and e-publications and associated websites. Selected examples include:

- National Institute of Mental Health (NIMH) website, affiliated institutes, programs, centers, websites, and publications (electronic and print)
- National Institute on Alcoholism and Alcohol Abuse (NIAAA) website, affiliated institutes, programs and centers, and websites and publications (electronic and print)
- National Institute on Drug Abuse (NIDA) website, affiliated institutes, centers, programs and websites, and publications (electronic and print)
- Canadian Centre on Substance Abuse (CCSA), affiliated programs and publications (electronic and print)
- National Center on Addiction and Substance Abuse at Columbia University (NCASACU), programs and publications (electronic and print)

3. Journals, magazines, societies, and associated websites. Selected examples include:

- *Psychology Today*
- *Scientific American*
- *Scientific American Mind*

As a practical matter, in researching particular topics electronically in psychopharmacology/ psychopharmacotherapy, the logical rule—as with everything else—is to search for topic(s), keyword(s), and the like on a search engine, then to narrow the search with entries given by the search engine. An important factor to keep in mind here is the reliability, accuracy, and quality of the source: Sources from (1) and (2)—above—are considered more reliable than those in (3), generally. Those in (3), in turn, are generally considered more reliable than personal blogs, newsletters, product websites, company websites, and the like.

Part IV
Synthesis and Conclusions

Chapter 13
Synthesis and Conclusions

To reiterate (from the first section of Chap. 3, "Antianxiety Agents"):

> A 38-year-old woman from the suburbs consulted her primary care physician assistant (PA) with complaints of severe tension and anxiety, insomnia, overeating, stage fright, and a pervasive sense of dread and foreboding. After interviewing and examining the patient, the PA determined that there was no obvious pathophysiologic basis for the patient's anxiety and prescribed a sedating (hypnotic) benzodiazepine, estazolam (Prosom®) for her. He instructed her to keep a daily mood diary, to call the practice before the next scheduled appointment and to return for a follow-up visit in two weeks.
>
> The patient returned as scheduled, appearing calmer, well-rested, energetic, and with a five-pound weight loss. She told the PA "Ever since I started giving the medication to my husband, I've felt 1000% better. Thank you so much."

Although intended as a fairly lame joke, this "case" actually illustrates a number of important clinical points which have been emphasized from the beginning and throughout this *Primer*. These points include:

- Proper diagnosis (Anxiety, in this case.)
- Clinically indicated medication (Benzodiazepine, in this case.)
- Use of other treatment modalities (Giving the medication to the patient's husband, in this case, "couples therapy," in a sense. Not a conventional approach!)
- Awareness of compliance/adherence factors (Concerning the husband in this case!)
- Awareness of the need for follow-up and proper interpretation of manifestational criteria—Epidemiologic Triangle model—symptoms ("…calmer, well-rested, energetic," in this case)
- Follow-up is obviously essential, especially for expected changes in patients'/clients' conditions (This is unlike the situation in which a stable chronic condition—e.g., schizophrenia; hypertension—can be monitored "from a distance," to coin the phrase, every 2–3 months.)

These points bring to mind other technical points and caveats which are summarized in Table 13.1.

© The Author(s), under exclusive license to Springer Nature
Switzerland AG 2022
D. P. Greenfield, *Psychopharmacology for Nonpsychiatrists*,
https://doi.org/10.1007/978-3-030-82507-2_13

Table 13.1 Important points in clinical psychopharmacotherapy

The use of psychopharmacological agents for given psychiatric disorders should be based on the best available clinical evidence.
Psychopharmacology should be combined, when appropriate, with evidence-based psychosocial and psychotherapeutic modalities in order to enhance medication adherence, reduce symptom burden and relapse, and increase function.
The choice of psychopharmacological agent is based on multiple factors, including evidence for efficacy, side effects, desirable secondary pharmacodynamics effects, routes of administration, drug–drug interactions, medical and psychiatric comorbidities, and personal and family history of medication response.
There is tremendous inter- and intra-individual variation in response to psychotropic medications.
If a patient does not respond to one drug in a given class, it does not mean that they will not respond to another drug from the same class.
In general, drugs that are approved for specific disorders are equally efficacious and differ primarily in terms of pharmacokinetics, adverse-effect profiles, and drug–drug interactions. The most notable exception to this rule is clozapine, which has unique efficacy for treatment-refractory schizophrenia.
When possible, minimize polypharmacy, which increases the risk for medication toxicity and drug-drug interactions.
Concerning drug–drug interactions (CYP-450 cytochrome enzyme oxidase systems), decreasing or increasing the doses of the necessary psychotropic medications should always be taken into account where potentially interactive drugs of any doses are administered which could increase or decrease the effective dose level of other drugs the patient/client is taking. Charts, tables, patient package insert (PPI) data, electronic databases, and other sources are readily available for this information.

Adapted from Hales et al. (2014)

All of the foregoing assumes that the prescriber is actually going to prescribe an "Anti-Agent" (psychotropic) of some sort, often with recommendations for accompanying psychotherapy/counseling of some sort, based at least in part on the presenting patient's/client's "chief complaint," symptomatology, and history. In fact, why bother to be able to prescribe—to undergo the time, effort, expense, and the like to become qualified to prescribe these "Anti-Agents" and other medications—if not intending and expecting to do just that? The answer to this logical question is central to this last part of this book.

In the words of Dr. Allen Frances, "The easiest and most mindless part of psychiatry is prescribing meds: be good at it, but not limited by it" (*Psychiatric Times*, October 2019). That prescribing of psychotropic medications has skyrocketed in the past 40-plus years is axiomatic, in part because, as the English writer and philosopher, Aldous Huxley, put it: "Medical science has made such tremendous progress that there is hardly a healthy human left;" in part because of the dramatic increase in practitioners with prescribing authority; in part because of what Dr. Frances calls "diagnostic inflation" through the *DSM-III, DSM-III-R, DSM-IV, DSM-IV-TR,* and currently *DSM-5*, and what Ethan Watters, in the title of his book *Crazy Like Us*, calls "The Globalization of the American Psyche"; in part because of the strong paradigm shift in medicine, in general, and psychiatry, in particular, toward evidence-based medicine in medicine and toward psychopharmacology and what is called "medication management" of symptoms in psychiatric practice and research; in part because of the dearth of prescribing mental health professionals in society who could treat patients/clients with modalities other than or in addition to psychopharmacotherapy; in part because of the convenience and rapidity (i.e., the perceived "quick fix") of psychopharmacotherapy and the public's demand for "quick fixes" to many of life's troubles ("Big Pharma" and the burgeoning created and existing consumer demand for relief from those troubles); and in part because of interactions among all of these various factors and trends.

But this *Primer* is, after all, a guide to psychopharmacology and not a wholesale detractor from that field. So, on balance, what beneficial observations and practices can be extracted from this book, both in summarizing the book (not as a "cookbook" for prescribing) and in encouraging sensible psychopharmacotherapeutic practice among the different types of prescribers who might use this book? In addition to the points made in Table 13.1 of this chapter, the following additional points and prescribing recommendations come to mind:

- **Trends change**. As described in the Preface of this book, the pendulum of what has been called "overprescribing" of psychotropic medications, or "polypharmacy," appears to be swinging away from that practice. "Deprescribing"— defined by the Bruyère Research Institute as "the planned and supervised process of dose reduction or stopping of medication that might be causing harm, or no longer be of benefit."— began recently in geriatric medicine and is moving into other areas and specialties in medicine, including psychiatry and psychopharmacotherapy. (Bruyère Deprescribing Research Team. What is deprescribing. In: deprescribing.org. 2020, June. https://deprescribing.org/what-is-deprescribing/)
- **Combination approaches** are generally recognized in the mental health professions—including those with prescribing authority—as producing better outcomes than either modality alone. In the case of psychopharmacotherapy plus something else, the role of that "something else" will likely become more appreciated by the prescribing professionals and the public as psychopharmacotherapy comes increasingly under the scrutiny of the "deprescribing" movement.
- As described early in Chap. 3 ("Antianxiety Agents"), the **research approach to psychiatric diagnoses has changed** dramatically in this country over about the past 10 years. If the "roots," or "causes" (in an epidemiologic sense) are determined in coming years, and psychopharmacotherapeutic intervention becomes specifically suited to those causes, then the role of medications will result in better treatment of symptomatology resulting from these causes, and better side effect profiles, presumably.
- Depending on the study, **"off-label prescribing"**—prescribing currently available medications for a clinical indication for which it has not received formal FDA approval—is common, conservatively estimated at 10 to 20% of all prescriptions; the practice is not considered per se illegal (Furey K, Wilkins

K. Prescribing 'Off-label:' what should a physician disclose? *AMA Journal of Ethics*. AMA; 2016). As frequently noted in this *Primer*, off-label prescribing of psychotropic medications permits greater flexibility and wider use of potentially useful agents for patients/clients.

So, in summary, this *Primer* is intended as a concise and practical guide to the nature, scope, and applications of psychopharmacotherapy, focusing on a classification system (i.e., the "Twenty Anti-s") based on manifestational criteria and symptomatology of patients/clients. The *Primer* is intended for a broad range of potential readers interested in the topic, as described in the Preface of the book.

This *Primer* is not intended as an encyclopedic, scholarly, or detailed "cookbook" of conventional psychopharmacology, as also first described in the Preface of the book. The fields of psychiatry, psychopharmacology, cognitive science, neuroscience, and related areas are awash with books, articles, reports, internet sources and information, symposium and meeting proceedings, electronic databases, and myriad other such sources. As mentioned in several places in this volume, the reader is referred to those sources for more detailed information about the vast topic of psychopharmacology.

The reader is also referred to the Selected References given at the end of the Preface of this *Primer* and to other references in various places in this book, for details of materials discussed in the various chapters. Some of these references provide such practical information as the available preparations of different agents, their doses and recommended dosing schedules, adverse ("side") effects, specific clinical indications, and the like.

Finally, I reiterate a point made early in this book: The success or failure of this *Primer* will depend on its usefulness to its readers. For that reason, I welcome feedback and suggestions to make this book as practical and useful as possible.

Please contact me with feedback and suggestions at dpgreenfieldmdpsychiatry@msn.com.

A Note on References

Rather than burdening the reader with excessive and detailed references and citations in this *Primer*, given below are particularly useful selected references. In addition, other specific references and citations will be given in parentheses throughout the *Primer*. For further information and details about any topics presented and discussed in this book, the interested reader is referred not only to the following list of selected references but also to applicable textbooks, monographs, electronic databases, print articles and materials, internet sources, and other applicable resources.

Selected References

- Black DW, Andreasen NC. Introductory textbook of psychiatry. 6th ed. American Psychiatric Publishing, Inc.; 2014. (A solid basic textbook of psychiatry.)
- Multiple Authors. Diagnostic and statistical manual of mental health disorders (*DSM-5*). 5th ed. American Psychiatry Association, Inc.; 2013. (This book is the controversial "bible" for primarily American and Canadian psychiatric diagnoses.)
- The comparable international work to the *DSM-5* is currently the 2019 International classification of diseases (*ICD-10*). 10th ed. World Health Organization. (The *ICD-11* was due for adoption in 2020.)
- Frances A. Saving normal: an insider's revolt against out-of-control psychiatric diagnosis, big pharma, and the medicalization of ordinary life. Harper Collins Publishers; 2013. (The subtitle says it all! See Chap. 4 in this *Primer*.)
- Ghaemi SN. Clinical psychopharmacology: principles and practice. Oxford University Press; 2019. (A scholarly, detailed, and lengthy overview of psycho-pharmacology, also covering social practice and research/methodologic aspects of the field.)
- Hales RE, Yudofsky ST, Roberts LW, editors, et al. The American Psychiatric Publishing textbook of psychiatry. 6th ed. American Psychiatric Publishing, Inc.; 2014. (A standard, detailed encyclopedic textbook tome, for reference. A seventh edition is available, copyright 2019, with updated coverage in a number of areas.)
- Harrington A. Mind fixers: psychiatry's troubled search for the biology of mental illness. W.W. Norton and Company; 2019. (A historical and scholarly review of the topic, including some of the same topics as *Saving Normal* listed above.)
- Puzantian T, Carlat DJ. Medication fact book for psychiatric practice. 6th ed. Carlat Publishing, LLC; 2020. (A very useful "cookbook" for psychotropic pre-scribing, conveniently organized and presented for the practitioner.)
- Watters E. Crazy like us: the globalization of the American psyche. Free Press; 2010. (Psychiatric diagnostic issues similar to those in *Saving Normal*, with an international focus.)
- Weil A. Mind over meds: know when drugs are necessary, when alternatives are better—and when to let your body heal on its own. Little, Brown and Company; 2017. (A balanced and holistic approach to pharmacology and psychopharma-cology by the popular "guru" of these fields.)

Selected Internet References

With the surfeit of internet resources, websites of all imaginable types and quality, and numerous related electronic sources of information and data, the reader, clinician, researcher, and member of the public—patient/client or not—may easily become confused about where to go and what to accept in learning psychopharmacology and psychopharmacotherapy. In this vein, a productive way to navigate the bewildering array of such sources consists of dividing them into several categories, viz.

1. Referreed ("peer-reviewed;" "juried") scientific, technical, and professional journals, newsletters, and the like, including e-journals, e-newsletters, and other open-source e-publications. Selected examples include:

   - *Journal of Clinical Psychopharmacology* (peer-reviewed independent professional journal)
   - *Experimental & Clinical Psychopharmacology* (peer-reviewed professional journal of the American Psychological Association)
   - *Journal of Psychopharmacology* (peer-reviewed professional journal of the British Association for Psychopharmacology)
   - *Psychopharmacology* (Berlin/Heidelberg; Springer Publications)

2. Government and academic/research institutions, publications and e-publications and associated websites. Selected examples include:

   - National Institute of Mental Health (NIMH) website, affiliated institutes, programs, centers, websites, and publications (electronic and print)
   - National Institute on Alcoholism and Alcohol Abuse (NIAAA) website, affiliated institutes, programs and centers, and websites and publications (electronic and print)
   - National Institute on Drug Abuse (NIDA) website, affiliated institutes, centers, programs and websites, and publications (electronic and print)
   - Canadian Centre on Substance Abuse (CCSA), affiliated programs and publications (electronic and print)
   - National Center on Addiction and Substance Abuse at Columbia University (NCASACU), programs and publications (electronic and print)

3. Journals, magazines, societies, and associated websites. Selected examples include:

   - *Psychology Today*
   - *Scientific American*
   - *Scientific American Mind*

As a practical matter, in researching particular topics electronically in psychopharmacology/ psychopharmacotherapy, the logical rule—as with everything else—is to search for topic(s), keyword(s), and the like on a search engine, then to narrow the search with entries given by the search engine. An important factor to keep in mind here is the reliability, accuracy, and quality of the source: Sources from (1) and (2)—above—are considered more reliable than those in (3), generally. Those in (3), in turn, are generally considered more reliable than personal blogs, newsletters, product websites, company websites, and the like.

Index

© The Editor(s) (if applicable) and The Author(s), under exclusive license to
Springer Nature Switzerland AG 2021
D. P. Greenfield, *Psychopharmacology for Non-Psychiatrists*,
https://doi.org/10.1007/978-3-030-82507-2

Printed in the United States
by Baker & Taylor Publisher Services